A M

# Authentic
# Foods

## Health Benefits of Whole Foods

## Facts, Recipes and More

## Bettina Zumdick
### Macrobiotic Counselor and Teacher

Nothing written in this book should be viewed as a substitute for competent medical care.

Cover photo by Bettina Zumdick

To place an order please call:
(413) 655-2751
or email:
**bettinazumdick@verizon.net**

**To My Son Sennin**
*whom I love and whose love and confidence in me made this book possible.*

# Contents

# Chapter 4:
## Sea Vegetables p. 129

# Chapter 5:
## About Myself p. 147

# Whole Grains

Most traditional diets are centered around whole, complex carbohydrates, such as whole grains.

Basically grains are small seeds that store source energy in a form that the body can burn without any toxic byproducts. By source energy I refer to the energy of the sun. They are able to capture the sun's energy through photosynthesis. One could refer to grain as crystallized sunlight. If you plant a seed of whole grain (non GMO), a new plant is going to arise. In other words it has a regenerating effect.

Whole grains are supplying us with carbohydrates. When talking about carbohydrates, it is actually not wise to throw all carbohydrates into the same pot, figuratively speaking. While there are many differentiating factors, two main types of dietary carbohydrates are important to distinguish:
- a) complex carbohydrates, also called starches which are basically many singular sugar molecules linked together to form a long, strand-like macromolecule and
- b) simple sugars such as fructose and glucose

occurring as singular sugar molecules and disaccharides such as maltose and sucrose, which occur as pairs of sugars.

Simple sugars, as in white cane sugar or fruits digest quickly and provide approximately 4 calories per gram. When we look at complex carbohydrates occurring naturally in their whole form, such as in whole brown rice they provide only about 1 calorie per gram only. This can translate into weight loss, if you are choosing complex carbohydrates as your source of carbohydrates.

Emphasizing a diet rich in whole foods, such as whole grains, vegetables, beans etc, means that the carbohydrates ingested are absorbed slowly, thus reducing the glucose load on the body within a given amount of time. This slow release of sugars into the body results in a control over the blood sugar and insulin. You may have heard of the glycemic index: the glycemic index is a measure of the effects of carbohydrates on bloodsugar levels. The higher the glycemic index of a particular food, the higher and more quickly the bloodsugar rises after ingestion of this food. While studying the glycemic index, scientists have found that the surface area of a food has the greatest impact on the glycemic index: the more refined and finely ground a food is, the higher the glycemic index is, or vice versa: the more whole and unrefined a food is, the lower the glycemic index tends to be. This indicates that there is a differentiation between whole grain kernels and whole grain flour: the glycemic index for whole wheat berries is much lower than the glycemic index of wheat bread or noodles for example. In a study arranged by the Harvard Medical School/Brigham and Women's Hospital, 74,000 women were followed over a 12 year period: weight gain was proportionally affected by the intake of refined grains and grain products[1].

Eating more whole foods and whole grains, allows the body to absorb the sugars from the complex carbohydrates very slowly but evenly over a longer period of time, because the long chains of complex carbohydrates take time to break down in our digestive process. The body will respond by releasing only a small amount of insulin into the blood stream. Reduced insulin levels are instrumental in helping people to loose weight, because insulin is a hormone that promotes obesity.

In any studies concluding that carbohydrates cause higher insulin levels, the carbohydrate content is almost exclusively refined carbohydrates.

---

[1] Relation between changes in intakes of dietary fiber and grain products and changes in weight and development of obesity among middle-aged women, American Journal of Clinical Nutrition, November 2003 vol. 78 no. 5 920-927

# Cardiovascular Benefits

A diet high in whole foods with complex carbohydrates is also decreasing the risk of cardiovascular diseases. Both cholesterol level and triglyceride levels can be drastically reduced. Triglycerides are the configuration in which fats are transported and stored in the body. There is an overall decrease of total cholesterol, with both HDL (high density lipoprotein) and LDL (low density lipoprotein) levels being reduced, but the greatest reduction is concerning 'bad cholesterol' levels or LDL levels. This translates to a decreased cardiovascular risk.

The American Heart Journal published a 3 year study of over 200 postmenopausal women with cardiovascular disease eating at least 6 servings of whole grains, including brown rice. The results clearly showed signs of slowing progression of artherosclerosis and stenosis (the constricting of the diameter in the arterial passages)[2].
Consumption of fiber from fruits, vegetables and refined grains was not linked with a slowing progression of cardiovascular disease.

---

[2] Erkkila AT, Herrington DM, Mozaffarian D, Lichtenstein AH. Cereal fiber and whole-grain intake are associated with reduced progression of coronary-artery atherosclerosis in postmenopausal women with coronary artery disease. Am Heart J. 2005 Jul;150(1):94-101. 2005. PMID:16084154.

There are many various compounds that help slow the progression of cardiovascular disease, including the cholesterol lowing effects of the polyunsaturated fatty acids, a particular form of complex sugar, called oligosaccharide, plant sterols (plant steroid components) and saponins. The wide range of antioxidants available in whole grains are invaluable for their ability to prevent damage from free radicals to cholesterol, which seems to contribute significantly to the development of artherosclerosis.

Dietary fiber from whole grains and whole foods is scientifically linked to lowering the risk of a variety of gastrointestinal diseases, heart disease, colon cancer and diabetes.

Simultaneously it is improving overall health, as it promotes a sense of fullness while it expands in the stomach during digestion and thus will reduce occurrences of overeating.
I will discuss two main types of fiber:
a) soluble fiber – ('Benefiber' advertises this kind of fiber on TV)
b) insoluble fiber – (Metamucil is a well-known brand in the US for this kind of fiber)
Pectins and gums are examples of soluble fibers – they dissolve in water and then begin a jelling process. This kind of fiber content in whole foods helps to lower the cholesterol by binding in our intestines and discharging it through bowel movement.

Insoluble fiber means that this kind of fiber cannot dissolve in water. However, it adds bulk to our bowel movement to propel waste out more quickly and it scrapes the tiny hair-like coating of our intestines clean, so that less mucous and bio film is blocking absorption of nutrients into the body. Whole grains contain a substantial amount of insoluble fiber, mostly known as bran.

Research has shown that insoluble fiber can help prevent gallstones, as it normalizes an overproduction of bile acids (excessive production is known to contribute to gallstone formation), as well as lowering triglyceride levels in the blood[3].

In the process of digestion, dietary fiber (both kinds) slow the speed of sugar absorption into the bloodstream – and the process is further slowed by the fact that eating whole foods usually goes along with consuming more complex carbohydrates, which are slower to digest than simple sugars.

---

[3] Tsai CJ, Leitzmann MF, Willett WC, Giovannucci EL. Long-term intake of dietary fiber and decreased risk of cholecystectomy in women. Am J Gastroenterol. 2004 Jul;99(7):1364-70. 2004. PMID:15233680.

# Sugar and Hypoglycemia

Many individuals in their 30ies and older, eating a standard western diet, such as an American Standard or Eastern European Standard diet suffer from a condition that is called Hypoglycemia.

Hypoglycemia is indicating that the blood sugar of a person often is chronically low and therefore symptoms like fatigue, shakiness, headaches, depression and many others can arise. The underlying cause of Hypoglycemia is the beginning or more developed condition of constriction. Tightness especially in the middle region of the body, particularly in and around the pancreas area is common. It can be caused by consuming an overabundance of animal foods or the loss of a loved one, stress on the job and many situations similar to these examples or combinations thereof. This constriction or tightness induces a desire for stimulants, sugar, sweets, alcohol, sodas, sweetened tea or coffee, etc. as these energetically have an expansive effect and will in the short term help to offset the tension and relax the person. However, when ingesting these foods/drinks that are laden with sugars, a person's blood sugar level tends to sky rocket for a short time and then drop precariously. While the blood sugar level is high one feels great, and as soon as it drops, life seems a misery. This emotional rollercoaster dynamic is played out by many people in this world on a daily basis, most people feeling the lull around early afternoon – when they start craving the mid-afternoon snack – perhaps a Danish or doughnut to intuitively prevent the blood sugar level from bottoming out.

If the solar plexus is tight or someone is suffering from hypoglycemia on a regular basis, this condition usually goes along with a belief of a constricting nature: the belief of not being good enough, being less than others and not deserving - or at least in some way switching back and forth between believing to be better than others and at other times being not good enough. And when we believe somehow that we are not good enough or that we are not enough, we also believe at some core level that there is 'not enough'. For example, the belief that there is not enough love is very common, and then we fill the gap or lack of love with sweets. Or perhaps a belief like lacking empowerment and eating sweets to cover up the feelings of victim hood and martyrdom or believing there is not enough time to do that which brings us joy and passion, so again we replace real joys and passion with sweets.

Let us say that somebody has hypoglycemia and regularly eats strong sweets to relax the middle area - and many people are actually not aware how much sugar they are eating when choosing to eat pastries, prepared foods, canned food and some condiments like ketchup. Let me tell you – it is a lot – the yearly average consumption of sugar per person in the US is approximately 150 lbs. In the long run this dietary pattern can turn into Diabetes or other diseases or problems may arise depending on the person's constitution and physical condition. A person who likes to have a candy in their mouth all the time, will quickly decay their teeth and especially ruining their gums – which may turn into gum disease, which if left unattended can cause inflammation throughout the body. Or if upbringing and social conditioning require a person to always be nice, it can at some point foster an explosion of emotion and even violence, because the person feels completely powerless and unable to channel her/his energy into living a meaningful life for her/him. For other people it can weaken their heart and at some point they might suffer from a 'broken heart' as in left ventricular prolapse where the contractive power of the heart is missing.

And we have to keep in mind that once we begin to eat strong sweets and stimulants on a regular basis, the body then wishes to make balance by craving foods with a more contractive power again such as salty foods, animal foods, hard baked foods or hard fried foods. This is allowing the body to constantly swing from pillar to post in terms of extreme contracting forces and extreme expanding forces switching places translating into a physically, emotionally and mentally exhausting rollercoaster ride.

Regular white or brown sugar is manufactured from the sugar cane plant. It naturally grows in the tropics and because of the way that it grows - long rods shooting upward - and the climate, the sugars derived from this plant have a strong rising effect. Plants naturally occurring in the tropical environment are well adjusted to their environment and the needs of the people eating them that live in that environment.

The refining process of sugar deprives it of all naturally occurring minerals and other phytonutrients – all refining processes of foods have the effect of manipulating our consciousness into disregarding the natural complexities of life and the natural connections with everything on earth.
It leaves us feeling separate and powerless. Eating whole foods on the other hand encourages more complex neural pathways in the brain and acknowledging the complexities of life, the intricate linked systems of connection from human to nature and spirit.

All of this is not to say that somebody in good health living in a colder climate will have a negative effect if he or she chooses to eat simple sugars occasionally. Only when we are talking about excess and when other underlying factors are at play, as well, will this create difficulty both physically and emotionally.

On a bio-chemical level, sugar (simple sugars like fruit sugar or cane sugar) stimulates the production of certain hormones including estrogen production. When the body receives the signal to produce certain hormones, it begins by producing more cholesterol, because cholesterol is a necessary building block for these hormones. This indicates that even when a person is eating a vegan diet, but incorporating a lot of sugar in their diet, their cholesterol levels can be high due to the sugar factor. This is not the case when consuming complex carbohydrates in the form of whole grains. Eating sugar in the long run can also have a negative and depleting effect on the immune function and spleen, which is part of the immune system.

The immune function is naturally nourished by downward, and concentrating energy dynamics. Especially and whole complex carbohydrates from grains and round, sweet vegetables have a very stabilizing effect on the immune function and middle organs.

The lymphatic system is an important part of the body's defense system. It is made up of a series of tubes called lymph vessels that branch out into all parts of the body.

Lymph vessels carry lymph – a watery liquid that contains white blood cells, called lymphocytes. A lymph node is a small bean shaped organ (in elbows, groin, neck, under arms) that filters lymph fluids. It filters out bacteria, virus and other foreign substances such as pollutants, parasites, toxins, and fungi. The lymph nodes may swell if the body is fighting an infection (for example a sore throat). As the body cells get nourished through the distribution of sustenance by the blood, at the same time, they release their waste into the intercellular liquid. Lymph capillaries collect the waste liquid and return it to the blood once filtered.

Due to modern eating and lifestyle, the liquid that enters the lymph system coming from the blood capillaries is not clear, but often fatty, cloudy and sticky. If intracellular liquid is sticky, and then is entering the lymph vessels, they become clogged and we feel tired, resulting in a desire to consume more stimulants and then feeling more tired after - a vicious cycle which is difficult to break. It simultaneously leaves us open for all kinds of diseases to take hold. Complex carbohydrates from grains and other natural plant food sources along with minerals from the same sources are strengthening the immune function and thus preventing many unnecessary illnesses.

# Metaphysical Understanding of Grains

The cooperative venture of nature, spirit and (wo-) man is exuberant, full of purposefulness. It exhibits the exhilaration of earthly and spiritual strength.

Grains, among other plants, remind us of cooperation:
- Cooperation among humans: becoming practicing idealists and thus being tolerant of the beliefs and ways of doing and being of others and while we are pursuing our own dreams and ideals, not being unkind to others in the process. Instead always anticipating and seeking our fellow (wo-) man's basic good intent and finding it, without and within.
- Cooperation between us and nature: nature is providing for us, and there is natural equilibrium in nature, however when we exploit the planet we simultaneously pull the rug out from underneath us and our descendents.
- Cooperation between us and spirit: without consciousness matter would not be in this universe. Consciousness gives matter reality and existence and thus consciousness or spirit sings through all of nature and even the void is full of vibrant vitality.

Have you seen fields of grain growing?

In Germany, where I grew up, mostly barley, wheat and rye fields were planted each year. I have most fond memories of watching the blue ethereal tone of rye fields as they matured during the spring and summer. The color is quite otherworldly and beautiful; it always made me feel calm and peaceful.

In grains the seed and the fruit are one. In fruits like apples for example, the seed is a separate unit within the fruit. This conjunction of fruit and seed being one has a more unifying effect. The source of power within and without comes always from unity. For example, let us look at a person who wishes to stop smoking: there is a part of the personality who wishes to continue smoking and there is the part that wishes to stop. These different factions within the personality make it difficult to stop smoking. By aligning the different factions of the personality into a unified front, this person can much more easily stop smoking.

If you have a garden space, consider incorporating growing your favorite kind of grain from heirloom seeds – all traditional cultures were aware that an area of grains planted (even just 1 square yard) is acting like an invisible boundary to keep negative influences away from the person who plants and tends to the grains with love, while their positive influence on a person's psychological structure help to balance and center a person. Grains emit a frequency or aura, which can strongly influence humans or any living being for that matter. If a person has a tendency to enumerate and focus on their failures, then the frequency of grains will bring in vibrations of rejoicing in one's accomplishments and one's positive characters. When all doors of thoughts seems to result in a dead end, the frequency of grains gently reminds us to trust that there is more in life than we can logically deduce and to let go of our mental distress. Grains can also help us when seeming unsolvable situations are arising. It allows us to rise to a higher vantage point from which we have a greater perspective and we can see and understand both ends of the spectrum, and thus we are able to embrace the paradox.

Most grains grow on a thin stalk, and at the upper most portion the seeds with the tassels are attached. Initially, when the plant is young the tassels reach right up towards the heavens, and as the plant matures, the seed heads become heavier and bend downwards a little. Through the roots the plant takes the physical nutrients from the soil and at the other end of the plant, the tassels function like human hair or antennae, picking up heaven's energy or the energy of the celestial bodies. Grains (as well as all other plants growing outside in nature) are continuously aware of the energies they are picking up from their surroundings and the celestial bodies. Also, when grains are imbued with a specific intent, such as becoming aware of your connection with your ancestors or growing to alleviate a disease that the person may have, they will with all their might pursue this line of exploration for the benefit of the person continuously without interruption. Most humans on the other hand are generally bombarded by the cacophony of voices from within and without, so that we are not able to pursue a line of thought continuously for more than a while (the duration of this 'while' varies depending on practice).

# Brown Rice

Brown rice, which actually is not brown but cream or beige in color, is my favorite grain. Rice has always been a staple in our home when I grew up and it was the first dish I learnt to prepare, when I was 8 or 9 years old, because it always made me feel wonderful. It still does.

Brown rice is the whole grain intact; just the outer, protective, hard shell is removed in a process called hulling.

As the whole grain is intact, when we soak grains long enough, they will sprout, as they contain their essential life-force. White rice cannot sprout; it lacks life force because it does not contain the germ any longer which is the place where sprouting would be initiated.

When cooking whole grains (any variety) it is important to soak them for 6- 8 hours or overnight prior to the cooking process. This will ensure that each rice kernel or grain kernel is beginning the process of germination. During this process the actual nutritional values of the grains increases, so that more nutrients become available to us.

Dry brown rice kernels contain enzyme inhibitors, such as phytic acid, which allow the grains to remain intact in a dormant state for a very long time, until the outer conditions are suitable for developing into a new plant again. These enzyme inhibitors unfortunately have a suppressing effect on our digestive enzymatic process. We can only partially digest non-soaked grains, with most of the valuable phytonutrients being un-available. Soaking will deactivate the enzyme inhibitors resulting in greater nutritional value and digestibility when eating the soaked and cooked rice.

Milling brown rice into white rice – also called polishing rice – destroys vast amount of phyto-nutrients and all the dietary fiber and essential fatty acids. Brown rice contains a fair amount of b-vitamins. 62% of vitamin B3 (Niacin) is lost in the process of milling, along with 85% of vitamin B1 (Thiamin) and 70% of vitamin B6, 70% of manganese, 58% of phosphorus, and 53% of iron. In the US white rice is required to be enriched with vitamin B1, vitamin B3 and iron. These added nutrients are not as effective as their natural cousins in the whole grain when consumed, and a lot of nutrients are actually lost in the process of milling that are not replaced at all[4].

Most of the nutritional value in grains is located in the outer layers (seed skins) of the grain kernel (not the outer protective hull). The inner most layer of the seed skins is called the aleurone layer. The aleurone layer along with the germ are bursting with health supporting nutrients, including essential fatty acids.

[4]  http://nutritiondata.self.com/facts/cereal-grains-and-pasta/5709/2 - brown rice

http://nutritiondata.self.com/facts/cereal-grains-and-pasta/5816/2 - white rice

Complete milling removes all of these layers, until only the carbohydrate sack in the center is left. In our western society a lot depends on the profit margin. The fatty acids contained in the aleurone layer and germ are volatile and can easily oxidize once exposed to the air. By removing these the shelf life of rice is extended – it won't get rancid, which means the rice can still be sold years later, and still bring profit to the owner/corporation or company – unfortunately not the end consumers. I believe that it is not only wise but in the long run advantageous to make choices that not only profit one person or a few but most if not all people. The germ (working in conjunction with the rest of the grain) contains the life force of the plant, it is like the embryo. The carbohydrate center of the grain could be viewed as the placenta, to feed the new growth of the plant when beginning to sprout. Milling rice or any grain for that matter, can be compared to throwing out the baby with the bathwater.

Rice is a good source of three trace minerals: manganese, selenium, and magnesium.

Manganese is significant for many varied purposes in the body's functioning: it is involved in the production of energy from carbohydrates and proteins; it plays a role in the synthesis of fatty acids (membranes in the body need fatty acids, as well as the nervous system). Also, the body requires manganese when producing cholesterol for the purpose of manufacturing sex hormones.

Manganese is a building block in the body's manufacturing process of Superoxide Dismutase enzymes (SOD's).

Superoxide Dismutase enzymes are found in brown rice, as well as inside the human body's mitochondria (the energy facilities inside most cells). SOD's are antioxidants, which prevent free radicals from becoming active. Free radicals can wreak havoc by fragmenting DNA, oxidizing fats or denaturing enzymes. SOD's are used to treat cataracts, arthritis and premature aging. Eating brown rice on a regular basis will help to prevent these diseases or reduce their negative effects.

Selenium, another trace mineral found in brown rice, is known for its ability to reduce the risk of colon cancer by inducing DNA repair, suppressing the growth of cancer cells and inducing the self destruct sequence for cancer cells. Thyroid hormone metabolism, antioxidant defense mechanism and immune function are also boosted in the presence of this trace mineral.

Selenium is also a crucial ingredient in many other vital systems in the body, including working with vitamin E for the prevention of cancer, heart disease and reducing symptoms of pain and inflammation regarding rheumatoid arthritis[5].

---

[5]

http://www.whfoods.com/genpage.php?tname=nutrientprofile&dbid=1
35

Brown rice contains a substantial amount of magnesium. Magnesium is an important part of our body structure, as two thirds of magnesium are embedded in our bones. Furthermore, magnesium can assist in preventing or abbreviating and reducing the severity of asthma, lowering high blood pressure and cutting back on the frequency of migraine headaches, as well as improving the odds of having a heart attack or stroke.[6]

Rice contains an enzyme, called glutathione peroxidase, which is known to reduce excess mucus, boost the respiratory function and helps to detoxify the body by disarming toxic molecules in the blood by passing through the liver where this enzyme is actively doing its work. Many other substances found in brown rice and other whole grains will also actively help with anti-inflammatory effects, the most known of these substances are the omega 3 fatty acids, magnesium and vitamin E.

Scientific studies try to analyze their objects of interest by dissecting them. Unfortunately, this mosaic separation and isolation into specific nutrients looses the greater perspective of the harmoniously orchestrated composition of phytonutrients working together. Yes, we can glean a lot from the scientific approach, but important details may be lost, even when looking at specifics.

---

[6] http://nutritiondata.self.com/facts/cereal-grains-and-pasta/5709/2

You have heard how fiber in the diet lowers the risk of colon cancer. Nevertheless it is important to differentiate: a fiber supplement may not be as effective as eating a whole grain. The phytonutrients from whole grains assist the body in a complex and multifaceted dance of health promoting steps that cannot be duplicated by a fiber supplement.

Most often researcher only measure the 'free' forms of phytonutrients with antioxidant power, as these are easily accessible for our bodies and get absorbed directly into our bloodstream. However, the 'bound' form of these nutrients also exist, but they are not studied in detail, because the accessibility of these nutrients depends on the availability of a healthy intestinal flora. The intestinal bacteria will release the phytonutrients from the walls of the plant cells during the digestive process.

Dr. Rui Hai Liu of the Cornell University has determined that phenolics, a group of powerful antioxidants widely studied in fruits and vegetables (apple, red grapes, broccoli and spinach), is available in its 'free' form up to 76%, whereas in grains such as brown rice it is available in 'free' form only about 1% and the rest of the 99% of phenolics are available in 'bound' form[7].

[7] Kafui Kwami Adom and Rui Hai Liu, Institute of Comparative and Environmental Toxicology and Department of Food Science, Cornell University, Stocking Hall, Ithaca, NY 14853-7201, J. Agric. Food Chem. 2002, 50 (21), pp 6182-6187 DOI: 10.1021/jf0205099 web publication: Aug. 31, 2002

You may have heard of catechins, quercetin, lignans, curcumin or ellagic acid – all of these are placed in the category of phenolics. If your digestive system is healthy and your digestive flora in good order then your body can easily disengage these phytonutrients from the plant cells via the intestinal bacteria and transport them into your bloodstream. Another way to ensure the best possible digestion of grains is eating a small amount of traditionally long time fermented pickles with your grains, because the necessary bacteria for breaking down the 'bound' forms of phytonutrients are provided through the long pickling process.

Brown rice and other whole grains are significant sources of the polyphenolic substance called lignans. Plant lignans are transformed into mammalian lignans through the digestive process. They can act both as phytoestrogens and antioxidants. Phytoestrogens means that lignans are capable of binding to estrogen receptors in the body and thus preventing cancer promoting effects of estrogen on the body (such as breast tissue) or other estrogen-sensitive cancers. The antioxidant power of lignans plays a role in many other health related functions, including the prevention of cardiovascular disease.

The FDA allows foods that contain at least 51% whole grains by weight (and are also low in fat, saturated fat, and cholesterol) to be labeled with a health claim stating consumption is linked to lower risk of heart disease and certain cancers. And newer research has shown that 2 – 3 serving of whole grains daily will also reduce the risk of type 2 diabetes. (van Dam RM, Hu FB, *Diabetes Care*)[8].

Please enjoy brown rice and many other whole grains on a regular basis. I have included some of my favorite recipes in the next section.

[8] Van Dam RM, Hu FB, Rosenberg L, Krishnan S, Palmer JR. Dietary calcium and magnesium, major food sources, and risk of type 2 diabetes in U.S. Black women. Diabetes Care. 2006 Oct; 29 (10): 2238-43. 2006. PMID: 17003299

# Whole Grain Recipes

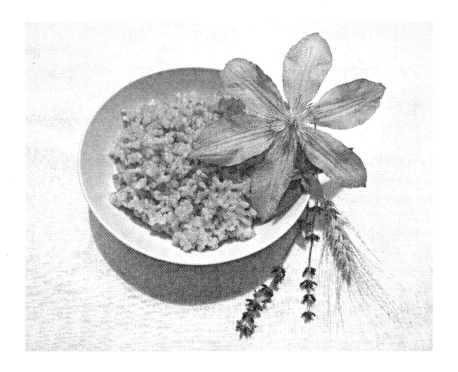

Brown Rice – Basic Recipe, see page 31

# Brown Rice – Basic Recipe

2 cups short, medium or long grain brown rice
4 cups of water
pinch of salt or a stamp size piece of kombu (sea vegetable), soaked

Soak 2 cups of washed and sorted brown rice in 4 cups of water for 24 hours. Place into a pot with a pinch of sea salt or a stamp size piece of kombu. Bring to a boil on a medium-high flame. When the water is boiling, cover and place a flame deflector underneath the pot (optional); then reduce the flame to low. Simmer for approximately 50 minutes. Turn off the flame, let the rice sit for a few minutes so that it will not stick to the bottom, and gently transfer to a wooden or ceramic bowl.

## Variations:
- 75 % brown rice cooked with one of the following: 25 % barley, millet, wheat, corn, etc.
- 75 % brown rice with chestnuts or almonds or sesame seeds or lotus seeds

# Barley Stew

½ cup of whole barley, sorted, washed and
soaked in 1 cup of water for 12 - 24 hours
6 dried shiitake mushrooms, soaked and finely sliced
1 inch piece of kombu, soaked and finely sliced
1 – 2 carrots cut into large chunks
4 inch piece of daikon, cut into chunks
4 inch piece of fresh lotus root, cut into chunks or ½
cup of dried lotus root, soaked and cut
1 – 2 onions, cut into chunks
1 cup fresh or frozen organic corn
½ cup finely chopped leeks
light barley miso  or chickpea miso
4 – 5 cups of water

Start cooking the barley in its soaking water in a soup
pot while cutting all of the other ingredients. Then
add all other ingredients in layers on top of the barley
in the following order: kombu, shiitake, onions, lotus,
carrots, daikon, corn. Add enough water to cover all
of the ingredients. Bring to a boil and turn down.
Simmer for 2 – 2.5 hours. Add water if needed. When
the barley is soft, season to taste with miso and add
finely chopped leeks for garnish.

# Rice with Spelt

1 ½ cups short grain brown rice, washed and soaked
12 – 24 hours in 2 cups of water
½ cup Spelt Berries, washed and soaked 12 – 24
hours in 1 cup of water
pinch of salt
pressure cooker

Combine rice, spelt and soaking water in a pressure
cooker. Add a pinch of salt, cover and seal the
pressure cooker, then turn the heat on high and allow
the pot to come to full pressure. Reduce the heat to a
low flame next, place a flame deflector underneath
and simmer for 50 minutes. Remove the pressure
cooker from the stove. Let the pressure reduce
naturally, then open the pot and transfer the rice and
spelt into a serving bowl.

# Meditation Rice

2 cups short grain brown rice
3 cups of water for soaking and cooking
1 pinch of salt
6 dried shiitake mushrooms
3 inch strip of kombu
1 cup of dried daikon
¼ cup of finely sliced takuan (rice bran pickled
daikon)
soysauce or tamari

finely grated ginger, lemon juice or finely sliced
scallions for garnish

Soak sorted and washed brown rice for 12 – 24 hours
in a bowl.

Place the grain and the soaking water into a pressure
cooker, adding a pinch of salt. Close the lid and bring
up to pressure on a medium to high flame. When the
pressure is up, place a flame deflector underneath the
pot and reduce the flame to medium-low, just enough
to maintain the pressure. Cook for approximately 40
– 50 minutes.

Soak shiitake, kombu and dried daikon together in a
bowl in plenty of water.

Remove the pressure cooker from the flame after the
40 – 50 minutes of cooking time and let the pressure
reduce naturally. When the pressure is completely
reduced, remove the cover, and gently transfer the
cooked rice to a wooden bowl.

After soaking the shiitake, kombu and dried daikon
for 30 – 40 minutes remove all ingredients from the
soaking water. Save the soaking water. Set the
shiitake and kombu aside for use in other dishes.
Finely cut the dried daikon. Add a small amount of
soysauce  or tamari and a small amount of the saved
soaking water to the dried daikon. Add this mixture
to the hot rice. Garnish with scallions and/or ginger
or lemon.

# Noodle Salad with Ume-Tahini Dressing

8oz. udon or somen or Soba Noodles
½ c cucumber, sliced into thin halves
¼ c celery, sliced into thin diagonals
¼ c red onion, sliced into thin half rings
¼ c red radish, sliced into thin halfs
1 - 2 cups chickpeas, cooked

Cook, rinse and drain the noodles or pasta, and place in a mixing bowl. Blanch the Red Onion, Celery and Red Radish separately for approximately 1 minute. Add all the vegetables and the Chickpeas into the mixing bowl.

## Ume Tahini Dressing
2-4 umeboshi plums
3-4 TB roasted tahini
1-2 TB finely grated onion
1 TB finely chopped parsley, scallion, or chives
¾ c water

Remove the pits from the Umeboshi Plums, and place the pulp into the suribachi. Grind until smooth. Place the Tahini, grated Onion, and Scallions in the suribachi and puree with with the Umeboshi. Slowly add water to the suribachi, pureeing until smooth and creamy. Pour the dressing over the salad ingredients and mix thoroughly. Place in a serving dish and garnish.

# Cornbread Recipe

1 ½ cups Whole Wheat pastry flour
1 cup Yellow Cornmeal
2-3 teaspoons non-aluminum Baking Powder
½ teaspoon Salt
1/3 cup Corn Oil or Sesame Oil
1 – 1 ½ cups of Water or Ricemilk
½ cup fresh or frozen Corn Kernels

Preheat the oven at 350F. Mix all the dry ingredients in a bowl. Add oil and water or soymilk, stirring until mixture is smoothly blended. The batter should be slightly thick, but not stiff. Fold fresh or frozen Corn Kernels in at the end. Place batter in a lightly oiled 9 inch square baking dish and bake for 30 to 40 minutes or until the edges are golden brown.

# Japanese Style Noodles with Piquant Tofu

8 ounces somen noodles, cooked al dente
1 lb firm tofu, rinsed, drained and cut into ¼ inch thick slices
soysauce or tamari to taste
water
2 or 3 cloves of garlic, minced
1 tsp. fresh ginger juice
approximately 6 TB of arrowroot
½ cup sesame seeds
sesame oil
2 carrots, sliced into matchsticks

2 small onions, cut into thin half moons
¾ cup fresh lotus root, cut into thin half rounds
½ cup of snap peas or snow peas

Marinate the tofu in soysauce or tamari, water, minced garlic and ginger juice for 30 minutes. The color of the marinade should be medium to dark brown.

In the meantime, place the arrowroot powder on one plate and the sesame seeds on a second plate. After marinating the tofu, remove the tofu, and dip the slices into the arrowroot powder first, and sesame seeds next. Each tofu slice should be covered with arrowroot and sesame seeds.

Whisk 2 – 4 teaspoons of arrowroot powder (from tofu slices or fresh) into the leftover marinade.

Over medium heat, fry the sesame crusted tofu slices in the oil. Remove the fried tofu pieces from the pan, when the sesame seeds begin to release their fragrance and turn slightly more dark in color. The arrowroot powder will have become translucent and created a firm coating with the seeds at this point.

In a second skillet stir fry onions, carrots and lotus. When these vegetables are almost cooked, add snap peas, stir fry for 1 more minute. Next stir in all or some of the marinade until it thickens.

Gently mix the stir fried vegetables with the cooked noodles  and top with sesame crusted tofu slices and serve.

# Rice and Spelt Pilaf

1 cup brown rice
¼ cup spelt
3 large onions
1 ¾ - 2 cups of water
2 - 3 tablespoons sesame or olive oil
¾ teaspoon salt
finely chopped parsley


Wash rice and spelt.  Soak separately for 12 – 24 hours. After soaking, dry roast spelt in skillet until fragrant, saving the soaking water. Cut the onions into thin half moons and sauté the onions in the oil in a pressure cooker. When the onions are soft and translucent, add the rice, spelt and the soaking water, as well as the salt. Place the cover on the pressure cooker and bring up to pressure. Reduce the flame to medium-low, place a flame deflector under the cooker and cook for 50 minutes.
Remove the cooker from the flame and allow pressure to come down. Remove cover and serve with parsley garnish.

# Sauerkraut Sandwich

whole wheat or rye sourdough bread
tahini
avocado (ripe)
sauerkraut
lettuce leaves

Mash 1/3 of an avocado with a fork. Spread a thin layer of tahini over the entire surface of one slice of bread. Next place a lettuce leaf on top of the slice of bread with tahini. Spread the mashed avocado on top of the lettuce leaf and finally top it with sauerkraut. Cut in half diagonally or in smaller square or rectangular pieces and serve.

# Noodle Sushi

1 lb. soba or udon noodles, cooked and drained
1/3 lb. firm style tofu, cut into ¼ inch thick pieces)
sesame oil for frying
soysauce
rice syrup and/or maple syrup
blanched watercress
pickled shiso leaves
nori

Preparing the tofu:
Place approximately ½ inch of oil in a pan and heat. When the oil is hot, fry the tofu slices in the oil until golden brown, then turn and fry the other side until golden brown, as well. Remove the fried tofu slices from the oil and drain excess oil on brown paper towels. Place 1 inch of water into a saucepan and season with soy sauce and brown rice syrup or maple syrup for a salty, sweet flavor, then insert fried tofu pieces and bring to a boil. Cover and simmer for 10 to 15 minutes. Remove the pieces and allow to cool, then cut into strips.

Preparing sushi:
Place one sheet of nori on a sushi mat. Place the noodles onto to the nori, so that the noodles are parallel to the bamboo sticks of the sushi mat, covering almost the whole nori sheet except the top edge. Spread tofu strips, blanched watercress and shiso in one straight line across the width of the noodles. Roll up, slice and arrange on a platter.

# Lasagne

1 package Lasagne noodles (16 oz), boiled in salt water
10 inch by 14 inch casserole baking dish
tofu cream, see instructions below
2 cups seitan, cubed
1.5 cups black, pitted olives
carrot sauce, see instructions below

## Carrot Sauce

8 – 10 large carrots, cut into medium thick rounds
pinch of salt
umeboshi vinegar
soy sauce
2 large onions, finely sliced into half moon pieces
1.5 cups mushrooms, finely sliced
1 medium red pepper, finely diced, optional
2 – 4 cloves of garlic, minced
pepper, optional
olive oil

Place the carrots into a saucepan and almost cover with water. Add a pinch of salt, and bring to a boil. Reduce the flame to a medium-low and simmer for approximately 20 minutes.
Place carrots and most of the carrot cooking water into a blender and puree to a smooth, creamy consistency.
Heat olive oil in a skillet and sauté the garlic, onions and mushrooms for approximately 5 minutes. Add the red pepper and sauté until all ingredients are soft. Season with soy sauce and pepper to taste. Add the carrot puree to the sauté and season with umeboshi vinegar to taste.

## Tofu Cream

16 ounces firm tofu
1 – 2 tablespoons soy sauce
½ cup water

Blend the tofu with water and soy sauce until smooth.

## Assembly
Pre heat oven to 375 degrees Farenheit.

1. Place a small amount of the carrot sauce into the bottom of a (10 inch by 12 inch – 3 inch deep) casserole dish.
2. Place a layer of the lasagne noodles on top of carrot sauce.
3. Then place a layer of tofu cream on top of noodles.
4. Next spread a layer of carrot sauce on top of the tofu cream, followed by a sprinkling of olive slices and a small amount of seitan cubes.
Repeat steps 2 – 4 until almost all of the noodles and carrot sauce and all of the tofu cream, olives and seitan cubes are used up.
Add one more layer of lasagne noodles on top, covered by the remaining carrot sauce.
Cover the casserole dish with a fitting lid or aluminum foil, not touching the food.
Bake for approximately 20 - 30 minutes at 375 degrees Farenheit.
Remove from the oven and serve.

# Pierogi filled with Seitan, Cabbage and Onion

## Basic Noodle Dough for Pierogi
1 cup of whole wheat bread flour, sifted
1 cup of unbleached white flour
¾ teaspoon salt
2/3 cup of cold water

Place the flour and salt in a bowl and mix thoroughly. Slowly pour in the water and form into a spongy dough. Knead the dough for about 10 minutes until the dough has the consistency of an earlobe. Let it stand for approximately 20 to 30 minutes. Then roll the dough, stretching it a little more with each roll until it is almost paper-thin.
Cut out square or round pieces and add filling into the center of each square or circle, fold the dough around the filling and firmly seal the dough. Then steam or boil the pierogi for 5 – 7 minutes. Serve immediately.

## Seitan, Cabbage and Onion Filling
1 lb seitan, minced
1c onions, minced
1c cabbage, finely shredded
½ c mushrooms, diced (optional)
sesame oil (regular or toasted)
salt
soy sauce or tamari (optional)
ginger juice (optional)

Sautee the onions, cabbage and mushrooms in a small amount of oil with a pinch of salt. Simmer until soft, then mix the seitan in. Depending on how well or strong the seitan is seasoned, you may or may not wish to add soy sauce or tamari and ginger juice towards the end of cooking.

If the pierogi are served with a dipping sauce or in broth, the filling may be mild to moderate in taste.

# Millet Loaf

¾ cup millet, sorted and washed
2 ½ cups of water¼ teaspoon sea salt
1 - 3 teaspoons soy sauce (optional)
4 inch piece of leek, finely sliced
1 medium to large carrot, cut into matchsticks
roasted sesame butter (optional)
ume paste (optional)

Place millet, water, salt, leek and carrot into a pot and bring to a boil. Cover and simmer for approximately 10 minutes before adding the soy sauce. Simmer for another 20 minutes. Remove from the heat and place the cooked millet mixture into a glass or ceramic bread form. Firmly pack the millet mixture into the dish. Cover with a bamboo mat and set aside to allow to cool. When cool, transfer the molded millet mixture onto a wooden board or ceramic plate for cutting. Cut into ½ inch slices. If desired spread roasted sesame butter and a small amount of ume paste on each slice and top with finely chopped chives or scallions.

# Blueberry Tart with Cookie Crust

**Crust:**
1 cup unbleached white flour
¾ cup whole wheat pastry flour
1/8 teaspoon sea salt
¼ cup sunflower seed oil
½ cup maple syrup
½ teaspoon baking soda
½ teaspoon almond extract
½ teaspoon vanilla extract

Preheat the oven to 375 degrees Farenheit.
Lightly oil a tart pan or line with parchment paper.
In separate bowls, mix dry ingredients and wet
ingredients. Next, gently whisk the wet ingredients
into the dry mixture until the dough forms a ball.
Using a rolling pin, roll the dough out to
approximately 1/8 inch thickness. Transfer the dough
into the tart pan, cutting off excess dough around the
edges. Bake for 5 to 12 minutes or until the dough is
golden brown. Remove from the oven and set aside to
cool.

**Filling:**
2 cups apple juice, organic
pinch of salt
1 tablespoon agar flakes
1 tablespoon kuzu, diluted in 2 tablespoons of water
¼ cup rice syrup or maple syrup
½ pint fresh blueberries
fresh mint leaves for garnish

Place apple juice, salt, agar flakes and rice syrup in a saucepan. Turn on heat and bring to a boil. Stir occasionally and boil until agar flakes are dissolved. Add diluted kuzu, stirring constantly to prevent lumping. Simmer until thickened. Stir in blueberries. Remove from heat and pour over pre-baked crust. Refrigerate to set filling. Garnish with mint leaves.

# Apple Strudel with Vanilla Sauce

### Strudel dough recipe:
2 cups unbleached white flour or 1 cup unbleached white flour and 1 cup whole wheat bread flour
½ teaspoon salt
¼ cup olive oil
½ cup cold water

Combine flour and salt in a large bowl. Add the oil and mix until the flour is coated and has a pebble like consistency. Add water and knead until dough forms into a soft ball – it takes approximately 10 minutes of kneading – add a little more water if needed. Let the finished dough sit in a cool place for a minimum of ½ hour, then stretch dough out by pulling it from the center into all directions equally into a very thin layer. You can roll the dough, however a rolled dough is generally not as thin as a hand stretched dough.

### Apple filling
4 apples, peeled, cored and sliced
½ cup of slivered almonds

½ cup of raisins, soaked for 1 hour in warm or hot water
small amount of flour

Spread the apples, almonds, raisins and a dusting of flour evenly on the dough, leaving the edges of the pastry uncovered.  Roll the filled pastry into a log shape. Place the strudel on a parchment paper lined pastry sheet. Bake in a pre-heated 375 degrees oven for approximately 30 minutes or until the crust is golden brown. Remove the strudel from the oven. Serve warm or cold.

## Vanilla Sauce
2 cups rice-milk or soymilk (grain syrup sweetened)
2 tablespoons kuzu
small amount of water vanilla powder or liquid.

Heat the rice or soymilk and vanilla in a saucepan. Dilute kuzu in a small amount of cold water.

When the milk is hot, add the diluted kuzu slowly, while stirring constantly until the milk has a sauce like consistency.  Serve hot with the strudel.

# Beans and Bean Products

From the western perspective, beans are a valuable source of protein, fiber, fat and minerals. And beans in combination with whole grains will provide all the essential amino acids the body needs. Essential amino acids are protein building blocks that cannot be synthesized by the human body and therefore must be supplied via our food. Beans and bean products such as tofu and tempeh can replace the animal food portion in a meatless meal. The benefit of very little animal food or no animal food lies in the absence of saturated fats, which are well known factors for high cholesterol and heart disease. In fact beans and bean products work in our favor to lower cholesterol and reduce the risk of heart disease.

From an eastern perspective, beans are foods that strengthen our kidney and urinary function. In the English language one kind of bean is called kidney beans, which is a testament to the fact that even in western culture there is an association between beans and kidney/urinary function. Also, kidney energy governs bone function. Many beans contain valuable amounts of minerals, including iron, phosphate, copper, magnesium, manganese, potassium as well as many others. These minerals not only strengthen the body as a whole, but furthermore are important for strong bones, healthy bone marrow, strong teeth, hair and nails.

Beans and bean products help regulate sugar metabolism (slowing the absorption of sugars into the bloodstream), water metabolism (governing kidney and bladder function energetically) and fat metabolism in the body.

In terms of our blood fat, beans help to lower the cholesterol levels, including lowering levels of LDL cholesterol and lowering triglyceride levels because of their soluble and non-soluble fiber content. Whereas eating animal foods (except fish) will generally raise one's cholesterol and triglyceride levels.

I had spoken about dietary fiber in the whole grains section. Bean fiber is benefitting the human body in the same way as whole grain fiber: Dietary fiber is scientifically linked to lowering the risk of a variety of gastrointestinal diseases, heart disease, colon cancer and diabetes. Simultaneously, it is improving overall health, as it promotes a sense of fullness while it expands in the stomach during digestion and thus will reduce occurrences of overeating.

The two main types of fiber are soluble fiber and insoluble fiber. Pectins and gums are examples of soluble fibers – they dissolve in water and then begin a jelling process. This kind of fiber content in whole foods helps to lower the cholesterol by binding in our intestines and discharging it through bowel movement.

Insoluble fiber means, this kind of fiber cannot dissolve in water. However, it adds bulk to our bowl movement to propel waste out more quickly and it scrapes the tiny hair-like coating of our intestines clean, so that less mucous and bio film is blocking absorption of nutrients into the body. Whole beans contain a substantial amount of fiber, many of them containing in a half cup serving more than 50% of the daily value of recommended fiber. At least two thirds of the fiber in most beans is insoluble, which means that is passes basically unchanged through the majority of our digestive tract until it reaches the last part of the large intestine, the colon, where this fiber is being broken down by very specific bacteria into short chain fatty acids. These fatty acids can be absorbed by the cells that line our colon wall and can be used by these cells for energy. This boost in energy from the insoluble fiber content in beans, allows our colon cells to remain free of stagnating factors that potentially could induce problems in the colon, including colon cancer.

Research has shown that insoluble fiber can help prevent gallstones, as it normalizes an overproduction of bile acids (excessive production is known to contribute to gallstone formation), as well as lowering triglyceride levels in the blood.

In the process of digestion, dietary fiber (both kinds) slow the speed of sugar absorption into the bloodstream – and the process is further slowed by the fact that eating whole foods usually goes along with consuming more complex carbohydrates, which are slower to digest than simple sugars.

Aside from fiber as a valuable macronutrient for blood sugar regulation, protein is another important factor in helping to stabilize the flow of food through our intestines and regulating the blood sugar absorption.

Especially garbanzo beans, also called chickpeas, have shown in a study that health benefits such as improving the participants' control of blood sugar levels and insulin secretion can be obtained in a very short time – as short as one week of eating 1/3 cup of these beans per day. Another benefit of garbanzo beans seem to be their higher satiation levels, which translates into less desire for processed foods and snacks and thus less consumption of these foods.[9] I love chickpeas for exactly that reason: they are rich and satisfying and I don't feel hungry for a long period of time after eating them.

---

[9] Murty CM, Pittaway JK and Ball MJ. Chickpea supplementation in an Australian diet affects food choice, satiety and bowel health. Appetite. 2010 Apr;54(2):282-8. Epub 2009 Nov 27. 2010

Pittaway JK, Ahuja KDK, Robertson IK et al. Effects of a Controlled Diet Supplemented with Chickpeas on Serum Lipids, Glucose Tolerance, Satiety and Bowel Function. J. Am. Coll. Nutr., Aug 2007; 26: 334 - 340. 2007.
Pittaway JK, Robertson IK and Ball MJ. Chickpeas may influence fatty acid and fiber intake in an ad libitum diet, leading to small improvements in serum lipid profile and glycemic control. J Am Diet Assoc. 2008 Jun;108(6):1009-13. 2008

When we experience stress, our body systems get damaged by free radicals in a process that is akin to rust developing on metal (iron) objects. The body systems that may be damaged in the process include the cardiovascular system, the lungs, the nervous system and the immune function. Antioxidants like vitamin C, vitamin E, beta-carotene, minerals and antioxidant phyto-nutrients are available in plentiful amounts in beans and hence will prevent damage, even help repair cellular damage.

Minerals like manganese – a key antioxidant in the energy-producing mitochondria found inside most cells, are provided in excellent amounts in beans. Also calcium and many other minerals and trace minerals.

Rich in omega-3 fatty acids (alpha linolenic acid), beans contain valuable amounts of polyunsaturated fats, which translate into a great benefit for our cardiovascular system and all membranes of our body. All membranes are made up of fats. Saturated fats are solid at room temperature. Desaturated or unsaturated fats are liquid at room temperature. Thus the more un-saturated fats our membranes are made up of, the softer and more flexible our membranes (including our skin) are.

Homocysteine is a sulfur containing molecule that the body produces when it is supplied by sulfur containing amino acids from animal protein. It is known to damage artery walls if it accumulates in high levels in our blood. It is considered a risk factor for heart disease. When sufficient amount of folate (vitamin B 9) and vitamin B 6 are available in the body, homocysteine will be broken down into benign components. Beans contain good to excellent amounts of folate and other b vitamins to prevent damage from homocysteine.

Plenty of magnesium is absorbed into our system by eating beans. This improves the flow of oxygen and nutrients throughout our body.

Most beans are quick growing plants climbing up on a trellis or another support structure. Some of the American Indian Tribes have traditionally grown 3 plants together, called the 'Three Sisters': corn, beans and squash. The beans would use the corn plant as its support structure to grow and the squash would cover the ground between and around the bean and corn plants to prevent weeds from taking over.

In my experience plant food creates a very different feeling tone and energetic signature on your being, than animal food does. And, please understand that I am not judging one as better or worse than the other, however, for myself, I generally prefer the more easygoing, peaceful and harmonious energy of plants over the very high-strung energy of animal food. I also suggest that the eating of animal foods also focuses the physical mechanism in the physical system, which can be of benefit, especially for hard physical labor. However, if you are in search of developing inner abilities, like intuition and flexibility of focus in consciousness for spiritual purposes, then

I would recommend moderation of intake of animal food.

Large studies have shown that meat-eating people are less healthy than large groups of people who avoid eating meat. Much higher rates of arthritis, colon cancer, hypertension, diabetes, ischemic heart disease, obesity and prostate cancer are found in animal food eating populations[10]. If you wish to decrease you risk, substituting beef, pork, poultry and other animal food products with beans and bean products is very effective and health benefitting. Another reason I cannot condone animal food eating is the inhumane ways we raise most of our animals meant for slaughter and the sustenance of our bodies. The animals are not granted basic quality of life, because profit margin is the most important aspect in our society. The lack of quality of life for these animals very much impacts their hormonal systems and thus all their body systems in a negative way, along with the well known fact of antibiotic and hormone use the animals are treated with.

---

[10] Fraser GE. Associations between diet and cancer, ischemic heart disease, and all-cause mortality in non-Hispanic white California Seventh-day Adventists. Am J Clin Nutr 1999; 70(suppl): 532S-8S.
Key TJ, et al. Mortality in vegetarians and nonvegetarians: detailed findings from a collaborative analysis of 5 prospective studies. Am J Clin Nutr 1999; 70(suppl): 516S-24S

Regularly consuming animal foods from animals, who during their life span were not allowed to enjoy life, may have an emotionally depressing and/or upsetting effect on humans.

# Vitamin B12

There is one aspect beans and bean products cannot provide for us nutritionally compared to animal food: vitamin B 12. Generally speaking it is difficult to find equivalent and sufficient amounts of vitamin B 12 in plant foods in general. The Recommended Dietary Allowance (RDA) for vitamin B 12 is 1 microgram daily. However, it is also well known that the liver can store vitamin B 12 for several years. More research has to be done in this area, because considering that vast populations in India and other countries are life long vegan and yet are not vitamin B 12 deficient indicates that perhaps certain bacterial cultures (perhaps ingested when eating live pickles) living in the intestines are able to produce and provide a person with vitamin B 12.

If you are concerned about vitamin B 12 deficiency, I would suggest that wild caught, and environmentally friendly caught fish from pristine waters, which contains virtually no or very little saturated fats, is one of the better options in terms of animal food eating and can provide us with vitamin B 12. One fillet of wild caught cod (20 ounces) contains between 2 – 4 micrograms of vitamin B 12. One can of wild caught sardines (3.75 ounces) contains 8.2

micrograms of vitamin B 12. Vitamin B 12 and folate supplements are also an option, as well as other animal foods. Vitamin B 12 is not heat sensitive, so will not be destroyed through cooking processes.

Long term Vitamin B 12 deficiency can cause permanent damage to the nervous system and other functions of the body. Symptoms can take many forms and are difficult to discern, unless a medical test is performed.

# Soybeans and Soybean Products

Soybeans in their whole form have long been recognized for their high protein content with many health benefits, including its anti-cancer properties. However, I am sure everybody has also heard controversial news about soy and soy protein: GMO is one aspect of the controversy, the processing of soybeans into certain non-natural soybean products is another aspect: soybeans are processed with solvents to create soybean oil for cooking or processed foods (the residue of the solvents remaining in the oil and the solid soy bean mixture) and the left over mixture is washed with water to manufacture soy protein concentrate for TVP (textured soy protein). This process creates a soy product that is very different from the whole soybean or naturally processed soybeans and retains very little if any of its health benefits.

Naturally processed or fermented soybean products

from organically grown soybeans, such as tofu, tempeh, or natto can be enjoyed by most people in good health several times per week. For estrogen sensitive cancers, such as breast or ovarian cancer, it may be best to avoid all soybeans and soybean products, as soybeans are high in phytoestrogen. However, a 2 or more years fermented miso containing soybeans, is different: during the prolonged fermentation time usually with salt, a grain and koji (a fermentation starter) the individual components of the beans and grains break down to such a degree that new substances are formed. This means that the phytoestrogens are broken down as well and will not interact with the body's receptors for estrogen.

Tofu is a soybean product made from curdled soymilk. The ingredients of a good quality tofu should only be: soybeans (preferably organic), water and magnesium chloride (sometimes also referred to as nigari). Calcium chloride is sometimes used instead of sodium chloride. In my opinion, this kind of tofu is like gypsum and is not easily digested. Sometimes also lemon juice is used to curdle the soymilk. Lemon juice is very cooling, and soybeans are very fatty, so we are creating a cooling fat, which has a tightening effect. Thus I would generally recommend tofu made with magnesium chloride, not the other varieties.

Tofu has a strong cooling effect on the body, which is great in the summer time to cool the body down. However if a person suffers from weak circulation and cold hands and feet often, it may be best to minimize tofu consumption or avoid it altogether.

Tempeh is a naturally fermented soybean product originating in Indonesia. The American version of tempeh is very much like a beef burger, dense and heavy. Traditional tempeh is fluffy and light, with lots of airy mold growing between the halved bean pieces. If you have the chance to taste the traditional kind - please do; it is very delicious. Tempeh is not ready to eat when you buy it – the beans are not fully cooked nor completely fermented during the fermentation stage. When you buy tempeh, it is best to cook it for approximately 30 minutes before consuming it.

Natto is another naturally fermented item – most available and popular in Japan. If you don't like strong smelling cheeses like blue cheese, then this may not be for you. Natto's texture is also very unusual: it is very slimy and stringy, like cooked cheese on a pizza. It is one of my favorite foods: when prepared with just a little soysauce, ginger juice and scallions, eaten with freshly cooked brown rice and nori (a seaweed) it is most satisfying for me.

When I was pregnant with my son, I craved natto and could easily eat two 6 oz containers in one sitting. I believe that the extra fat in soybeans and the specific bacteria helped me with adequate nutrition. However, when I ate too much natto, I would feel spaced out.

After my son was born, and beginning to eat more solid foods, I was surprised to find that he also loved natto.

When prepared well, all of these soybean products can taste very satisfying and delicious.

Especially tofu can be prepared in such a variety of ways, so that it can be enjoyed all year round – cooling in the summer time and warming, rich dishes in the winter time.

# Bean Preparation – General Info

The first step in bean preparation is sorting your dry beans – beans sometimes contain small rocks and dirt piles or other debris that may damage your teeth or enjoyment of eating the beans. Also remove any broken or damaged beans. The damaged beans become rancid rather quickly because of the higher content of fat in beans.

Next, wash the beans carefully, then soaking them in plenty of fresh water (for each cup of beans use 2 – 3 cups of water) for 12 – 24 hours. The soaking process reduces cooking time and makes beans easier to digest: specific flatulence causing sugars (such as stachyose and other oligosaccarides) may be reduced during the soaking process along with a reduction of the phytic acid and enzyme inhibitors found in dry beans, which decreases mineral absorption from foods in the intestines.

After the soaking process, discard the soaking water and rinse the beans with fresh water.

To cook beans, you may either choose a heavy pot, to cook on the stove or a pressure cooker. Stove top boiling may take between ¾ hour – 3 hours of cooking time depending on the kind of bean (small or large) and the age of the beans – older beans have dried out longer and thus take a much longer time to soften. Also the water quality and geographical area will influence cooking time: if your water contains a lot of minerals ('hard' water) it may slow the process of cooking, whereas 'soft' water allows beans to cook more quickly. Living at sea level versus up high in the mountains is another factor which determines cooking time. At sea level the air pressure is higher than at 12,000 feet, and the boiling temperature of water much higher at sea level than high in the mountains. A lower boiling temperature will prolong the proper cooking of beans.

Pressure cooking is a wonderful way to shorten cooking time – in my home chickpeas, when properly soaked will pressure cook in half an hour. Before I start the cooking process I usually add Kombu, a sea vegetable to the beans, which helps to soften them and also helps in making them more digestible.

Begin the cooking process by leaving the lid open while the beans are coming to a boil. Often a grey foam rises to the surface, that is best removed with a slotted spoon or a skimmer. Once no more foam is arising, I close the lid and turn the flame down low to simmer the beans slowly until they are fully cooked. It is best to season beans at the end of the cooking process usually with salt or other salty agents (sea vegetables are an exception) otherwise the beans remain hard.

Should you decide that cooking beans is too complicated, canned beans are an option, and I would recommend Eden brand beans, as their cans do not contain BPA (bisphenol-A), an endocrine disrupter found in most cans available on the markets today. Instead they use natural oleoresin coming from plants such as pine and balsam fir, which does not negatively impact our hormone function.

# Bean and Bean Product Recipes

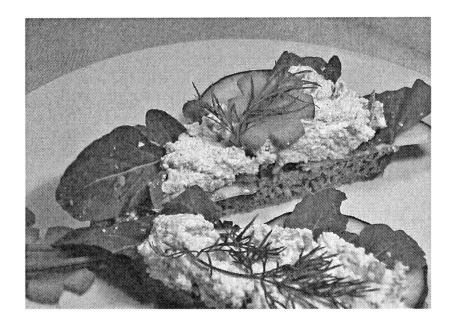

Tofu Patê Sandwich, see page 69

# Spicy White beans with Onions, Cabbage, Sauerkraut and Pepper

1 cup navy or great northern beans, soaked overnight
in 3 – 4 cups of water
2 cups onions, sliced into half moons
1 ½ cups sauerkraut, liquid squeezed out
2 cups green cabbage, finely sliced
2 – 3 tablespoons sesame oil
pepper to taste
1 piece of kombu, 1 inch long
sea salt to taste

Discard the bean soaking water and rinse the beans
in plenty of fresh water. Place the beans and the
kombu into a pot and cover with water –
approximately 1 inch of water above the bean level.
Bring to a boil with an open lid. Remove any grey
foam that may rise to the surface. Reduce to a
simmer, cover, and cook until the beans are 80%
done, adding water as needed.
Sauté the onions in the sesame oil until glassy.
Remove the beans from the cooking pot and place the
sautéed onions into the bottom of the bean pot, layer
the cabbage on top of the onions, then the beans with
their left over cooking liquid and as a final layer the
sauerkraut. Bring back up to a boil and simmer,
seasoning all the ingredients with pepper and salt,
simmer for another 10 minutes and serve hot or
warm.

# Tempeh Rueben

1 package tempeh (8oz.), sliced into thin strips
1 cup green cabbage, shredded
½ cup sauerkraut
½ lb. mochi, grated
soy sauce or tamari to taste
sesame oil
water
whole-wheat sourdough bread or pita pockets

Heat sesame oil in a skillet and brown the tempeh slices on both sides. Next, add enough water to cover the tempeh, along with a few drops of soy sauce or tamari, to taste  then layer the sauerkraut and cabbage on top and cover the skillet. Simmer for approximately 10 minutes; add water if needed. Remove the cover and place the grated mochi on top. Do not mix. Cover and cook until the mochi melts – the mochi will not melt if you leave the skillet uncovered!
Serve hot on whole-wheat sourdough bread or in whole wheat pita pockets.

# Tofu French Toast

16 ounces firm tofu, drained
whole-wheat sourdough bread, sliced
1 tablespoon soy sauce or tamari
½ cup water
sesame seed oil or sunflower seed oil
rice syrup or maple syrup


Blend the tofu with water and soy sauce or tamari in a blender until smooth. Place the blended tofu cream into a shallow, large bowl.

Heat enough oil in a griddle or shallow skillet to cover the bottom of the skillet. Take one slice of bread and coat both sides of the bread with the tofu cream. When the oil is hot, fry both sides of the tofu coated bread until slightly crispy. Repeat this process until all the tofu cream is used up.

Serve hot with rice syrup or maple syrup.


# Tofu filled Pierogi

### Basic Noodle Dough for Tofu filled Pierogi
1 cup of whole wheat bread flour, sifted
1 cup of unbleached white flour
¾ teaspoon salt
2/3 cup of cold water

Place the flour and salt in a bowl and mix thoroughly. Slowly pour in the water and form into a spongy dough. Knead the dough for about 10 minutes until the dough has the consistency of an earlobe. Let it stand for approximately 20 to 30 minutes. Then roll the dough, stretching it a little more with each roll until it is almost paper-thin.

Cut out square or round pieces and add tofu filling into the center of each square or circle, fold the dough around the tofu and firmly seal the dough. Then steam the pierogi for 5 – 7 minutes. Serve immediately.

## Tofu Filling for Pierogi
½ lb of tofu
1 teaspoon of soy sauce
½ teaspoon of ume paste
¼ teaspoon of shiso powder
½ teaspoon of nori flakes
1 tablespoon minced scallions
½ tablespoon of arrowroot powder

Puree tofu in a hand-food-mill.
Mix ume paste, shiso powder, nori flakes, scallions and arrowroot powder in a suribachi. Add pureed tofu to suribachi and mix well.
Use for fillings in pierogi or steamed tofu rolls, etc.

# Azuki Bean Mochi Delight

1 cup azuki beans, washed, sorted and soaked
overnight in 3 – 4 cups of water
1 stamp size piece of kombu
1 package mochi
1 pinch of sea salt
Rice syrup to taste

Boil azuki beans, inclusive of their soaking water, for
1 to 1 ½ hours or until they are soft. Add water if
needed. When the beans are soft, add salt and cut the
mochi into small squares. Add rice syrup to the beans
to taste, then place the mochi on top of the beans,
simmer until mochi has softened or melted. Serve
warm.


# Minestrone

1 cup of kidney beans (pre-soaked and cooked)
2 inch strip of kombu
1 - 2 onions, diced
½ cup carrot, diced
½ cup celery, diced
½ cup corn, fresh or frozen
½ cup whole wheat or brown rice rotini
6 dried shiitake, soaked and finely sliced
1 – 2 cloves garlic, minced
½ cup parsley, finely sliced
3 scallions, thinly sliced
sesame oil
approximately 6 cups of water

sea salt to taste

To wash and pre-soak beans: Sort through the beans, discarding any broken beans, stones, clumps of soil. Wash beans well and place into a bowl, adding water to cover and soaking for a minimum of 6 hours or overnight. After the soaking time discard the soaking water and add enough fresh water to cover the beans.

Place kombu into a pressure cooker. Add the beans and water. Bring the beans to a rapid boil and skim off any foam that may collect on top of the beans. Two to three skimmings will greatly reduce or eliminate gas producing matter.

Place the lid on the pressure cooker, bring to high pressure, then reduce flame to low. Pressure cook for 1 hour. Let the pressure reduce naturally and open the pot. Remove the kombu from the pot, dice it and return it into the beans.

Sautee the onions and minced garlic cloves in a soup pot. Next add water, beans, carrots, green beans and celery into the pot. Bring to a boil, then add the rotini. Cook until the vegetables and macaroni are cooked, but not overcooked. Add the parsley and salt to taste. Cook a few more minutes. Serve soup garnished with scallions.

# Tofu Patê Sandwich

½ pound firm tofu, drained
1 – 2 umeboshi plums
1 – 2 teaspoons grated onion
1 – 2 teaspoons celery, finely diced
1 teaspoon shredded carrot
Several slices of cucumber
Several tablespoons alfalfa or broccoli sprouts
Lettuce
Whole Grain Sourdough Bread

Place the umeboshi plums into a suribachi and puree to a smooth paste. Add the onion and tofu and puree to a smooth consistency. Add the celery and shredded carrot and a few drops of shoyu and mix well. Spread this mixture on sourdough bread slices. Top with cucumber slices, sprouts and lettuce and another slice of bread if desired.

# Vegetable Energetics

## Leafy Greens

Have you heard of chakras? Chakras are spiral- or wheel-like energy centers along the vertical axis of our body, created by the meeting of heaven's downward moving force and earth's upward moving force. There are seven main chakras in the body, and each of these has a different color associated with them. The color for the heart chakra is a vibrant emerald green. During the summer in our climate we are immersed in vibrant green colors from nature – lush green grass, various shades of greens from trees and bushes, shrubs, flowers, weeds and of course also leafy greens we eat. The reflection of the green spectrum of plants is very useful to the plants because they cannot absorb the green light. And green light for us is very beneficial as it has a therapeutic value for the human psyche.

And it is during our summers that I notice many people's hearts being more open, happier and more vibrant, as the green color reflecting everywhere is stimulating heart energy and heart centered living.

The green color reminds us that the universe actively loves itself and all of its parts. It is the miraculous principle of pleasure, which is an active, positive fueled energy that is rejoicing in itself and its own characteristics. Imagine yourself walking through a deciduous forest, the rays of sunlight filtering through the leaves, and just by allowing yourself to be immersed in this vibrant, emerald green sea of leaves, the love for yourself, others and the divine is being re-kindled. There is nothing that you have to do or achieve, just allow yourself to be.

Green is the energy of love, one of the greatest creative forces of all physical life. It operates in an almost leapfrog fashion, with great bursts of exuberance and vitality.

This greatest creative force does not dissipate. Instead it is re-created constantly in cycles, like the cycles of the seasons. With ever-new virgin energy arising in the springtime, each new sprout, each new plant is completely new and unique, utterly itself, innocent and vibrantly alive in the world and imbued with the miraculous principle of pleasure that propels life itself. And plants growing naturally and joyfully never question: should I grow a little more to the left or to the right? Should I have a different color? Whereas these are questions we might waste time on, instead of being ourselves and by being ourselves blessing ourselves and others simultaneously. When we consume naturally grown plants (in the soil and exposed to the celestial bodies), which are imbued with their natural joy and pleasure in themselves and in the universe, we receive this energy signature: first via our digestive system, and then it is transported into our cells and from our cells into our mind. Thus we are reminded of our natural being and natural joys and pleasures. What a lovely way to perpetuate and increase the joy of this world.

Leafy greens, like watercress, kale, collards, napa, bok choy and many more are available these days year round. And aside from the 'love and joy' factor, leafy greens are an important component in any diet because they provide quite a substantial amount of fiber, minerals, especially Calcium and if eaten raw or cooked less than 2 minutes, also significant amounts of Vitamin C.

Vitamin C is heat sensitive and will be destroyed when cooked longer than 2 minutes. Thus quickly steaming, quickly blanching, short sauté or pressed salads are better options for cooking methods of greens.

Leafy greens also contain chlorophyll, which is a compound that aids in producing healthy red blood cells. Our red blood cell molecules, called hemoglobin, have almost the same structure as a chlorophyll molecule: the only difference is that chlorophyll contains a magnesium atom in the center, whereas hemoglobin's center is graced by iron.

The various minerals in greens, such as calcium, iron and magnesium compounds, as well as many other trace minerals and other phyto-nutrients will help to neutralize acidities in our blood stream and our body as a whole. Furthermore they strengthen the immune function, because a lack of minerals results in a weak immune system.

Leafy greens are upward growing plants. Like trees or shrubs, they utilize carbon-dioxide and release oxygen into the air, thus breathing opposite of us or to say it more simply: they are providing oxygen for the human body (however, the greatest producers of oxygen for the planet comes from ocean phytoplankton). Photosynthesis is respiration in exact reverse. This function will help strengthen our respiratory system and body system as a whole, as oxygen needs to be distributed to all parts of our body for efficient functioning.

Our respiratory function also plays an important role in the body's ability to excrete waste, as well as governing our ability to speak. When we strengthen our excretory function through breathing, we simultaneously improve the function of another excretory function in our body: bowel movement.

The amount of fiber available in greens provides bulk for propelling stools through the digestive system more quickly and more regularly. These days we are bombarded with advertisements on TV and the internet about constipation relief medications. Obviously constipation has become a rampant problem in the modern world. Part of the problem is that our contemporary diets are devoid of most, if not almost all fiber, which would help our septic system (the digestive system). The fiber content in leafy greens expand in the stomach, creating a sensation of fullness thus preventing us from overeating, as well as lowering the transit time through the intestines.

According to the oriental understanding, the liver and gallbladder are classified as 'tree' energy (please refer to other books for more info, for example: 'Holistic Health Through Macrobiotics' by Michio Kushi and Edward Esko, Chapter 1, pp. 36) in the five transformation theory. This means that the liver's energy is upward and rising. Eating leafy greens as part of our daily diet, at least twice a day will ensure a happier and better functioning liver and gallbladder. The liver is one of the most important filters in the body. Its function is to detoxify along with being in charge of quite a lot of other functions, as well. The upward energy of leafy greens tremendously supports the multifaceted functions of the liver.

Greens are simply delicious. However, if you find greens too bland or tasteless, you may wish to prepare a dressing. One of my favorite dressing is pumpkinseed dressing.

## Steamed Greens

Steaming greens for a short time is a light and quick way to prepare greens. However this cooking method also has a somewhat drying effect, which means that it concentrates the flavor of the vegetable: naturally sweet tasting leafy green vegetables, such as napa or bok choy, become sweeter, and naturally strong tasting vegetables like dandelion greens or sometimes collard greens with a bitter flavor will become more bitter in taste.

Hence I would recommend using cooking methods like blanching or quick sauté for strong tasting vegetables, as their strong taste will be offset by these cooking methods. In other words the strong or sometimes bitter tasting components will be released through blanching into the cooking water or balanced through the oil in the process of a quick sauté.

Energetically, steaming is a very light cooking method when prepared in less than two minutes. The highly excited water molecules provide an activating effect for the vegetables. The inclination of this cooking method, however, is toward a more centering and calming effect, as the vegetables are not moving themselves.

## Blanched Greens

Blanching greens is a very different cooking method: we have vegetables cooking in plenty of boiling water, which means the vegetables are actively tumbling around in boiling water.
To retain vitamin C while blanching leafy greens, it is best to cook the greens less than two minutes, due to the easy destruction of Vitamin C through heat.

The active movement of the vegetables prepared this way accounts for a more dispersing and loosening effect. For example, imagine plaque build up in the arteries: it is an accumulation that is beginning to harden and becoming static and inflexible. This particular cooking method will help energetically to shake loose debris and dispose of the debris (hardening of the arteries) through the natural channels of cleansing the body.

Any systems of our body carrying or utilizing some form of liquid will be particularly positively impacted, as water is the medium for this cooking method. Thus stagnating accumulations that may have built up in the circulatory system (blood and blood vessels), the lymph system, carrying lymph liquid, and the urinary function, especially the kidneys can be cleansed and refreshed by this cooking method.

And remember that you can imbue a dish like this one with even more effective health, joy and vibrant properties by blessing the water with your strongest intention and wishes of these purposes. Water is particularly susceptible to carrying intention, as explicitly shown by the Masaru Emoto's book: ' The Hidden Messages in Water' - water reflects our consciousness or state of mind.

Sometimes I blanch leafy greens whole and cut them after cooking, while at other times I cut them before I begin the cooking process. Blanching whole leaves, like napa leaves or collard leaves, will retain more nutrients, because there are less areas which are open to leaching nutrients into the water. However, even if I blanch whole collard leaves or kale leaves, I most often trim the center vein out of the leaf, as the cooking time for the thick center vein takes a lot longer and if I were to wait for the center vein to be cooked properly, the leafy part will be overcooked. In other words, center veins along with the stems of most leafy greens have a longer cooking time and it is best to cook them separately from the leafy part.

And by the way, there are controversies about drinking the left over greens cooking water all the time or using it for soup stock daily, as some greens actually release some semi toxic components into the cooking water. Therefore it is best to discard the cooking water from leafy greens most often, especially from greens like kale and collards.

## Quickly Sautéed Greens

Quick sautéing is another preparation well suited for leafy greens, as well as other vegetables and vegetable combinations. A literal translation of the French word sautéing means jumping or skipping, which is what we are making the vegetables do – we have them jump and skip around in the skillet. Quick sauté indicates that we take very finely cut leafy vegetables, which we briefly stir fry in a small amount of good quality oil or water, until they are softened or wilted, but still retaining their vibrant green color.

As we all know, jumping and skipping has an activating effect on our bodies, and metaphorically speaking, eating sautéed leafy greens will thus have an activating effect on our bodily systems.

The combination of leafy, green vegetables (stimulating our lung function and ability to communicate) with this cooking method (activating) will have a doubly stimulating effect on our ability to communicate or being communicative and being socially active.

## Pseudo Cooking Methods: Pressed Salad

Ok, here we go: what is a pressed salad?

It has nothing to do with a regular lettuce salad, although lettuce may be one of the vegetables used in a pressed salad. A pressed salad is a pseudo cooking method, in which we take raw vegetables, cut them finely, mix and kneed them with salt or a salty seasoning solution such as ume vinegar or soy sauce and finally press the salted vegetable mixture, until the water is drawn out of the vegetables which may take 10 minutes to 4 hours, depending on the density of the vegetable, how finely we have cut (or grated) the vegetables and how much salt we have added.

Some people are misleadingly calling this a quick pickle – this is not a pickling method. Pickling suggests the presence of pro-biotic bacteria from the process of pickling. Four hours of pressing vegetables with salt in not enough to allow for any worth mentioning amount of pro-biotic bacteria to arise.

However, a pressed salad is a raw vegetable dish, thus all the heat sensitive nutrients are available in their entirety, including all the enzymes. By breaking down the vegetables in the process of pressing them with salt, they become more alkaline. This is helpful to keep our blood slightly alkaline, and the nutrients are easily accessible during the process of digestion. As the water content is removed during the process of pressing the vegetables with salt, eating a pressed salad has a less cooling effect than eating a completely raw salad.

Just think of eating a raw cucumber salad in the middle of winter, when the temperatures in this part of the country easily fall below zero degrees Fahrenheit. Unless you are eating a lot of animal food, which has a warming or heating effect, raw cucumber salad will leave you feeling cold or frozen. And it will take a lot of energy for the body to keep the body temperature within a normal range or to warm the body up to the appropriate temperature. When eating a pressed salad instead, it has a much less cooling effect, doesn't sit in the intestines for as long and thus is from an energetic perspective much more energy efficient – leaving more energy for extra brain excursions or other fun we might wish to engage in.

Pressed Salads are excellent during all seasons –

smaller amounts in the winter time and larger volume during the warmer seasons, generally speaking. However, when our body is too overheated from eating vast amounts of heavy animal foods, like heavy meats or a lot of heavier dairy products like cheese pizza, etc., increasing pressed salads even during the cooler seasons may be appropriate.

# Pickles

Fermentation or pickling is the conversion of carbohydrates to carbon dioxide and/or organic acids using yeasts or bacteria or a combination thereof, under anaerobic conditions.

Fermentation usually implies that the action of microorganisms is desirable, as opposed to spoilage, which gives us a stomach ache.

Fermentation is used in the leavening of bread, alcoholic beverages and for preservation techniques to create lactic acid in sour foods such as sauerkraut, kimchi, vinegar, yoghurt, miso or other pickled foods, as well as vinegar.

Lactic acid fermentation has been an essential part of healthy human diets throughout the world for thousands of years. It was primarily used as a way to preserve vegetables throughout the winter season and to retain the nutrients in the vegetables without the need for refrigeration. It is well known that sauerkraut was on board long ship voyages before refrigerators were available, because it prevented the sailors from experiencing the atrocious effects of scurvy – a vitamin C deficiency.

Producing raw, lactic acid fermented (or naturally fermented) pickles went out of favor with the advent of industrial food production. Lactic acid fermentation produces a variety of healthful substances, primarily lactic acid bacteria.

Many varieties of pickling methods exist, depending on the climate you live in. Pickling in four season climates is usually a process of mixing well washed vegetables, which may be sliced or grated as needed, with sea salt or a salt brine (a water and salt solution). The salt acts to draw out the juices, and is the selecting agent to allow only certain kinds of bacteria (salt loving bacteria) to become active and proliferate.

Similarly in our body, when our blood condition is slightly alkaline, only salt loving bacteria can thrive in our gut, also called beneficial bacteria or probiotics, however, when our blood condition becomes too acidic, then yeast bacteria such as candida can increase tremendously and lead to yeast infections and many other kinds of infections and health compromising conditions.

The vegetable-salt mixture for pickling is packed into fermentation vessels, such as glass jars or ceramic crock pots or wooden barrels and placed in a well ventilated, but relatively warm spot (best between 70 – 75 degrees Fahrenheit) for a certain period of time.

Long term pickles may need to ferment months or years before they are ready to eat, whereas short term pickles may only take a few days to ferment. The longer the fermentation, the more beneficial bacteria will have been produced.

# Benefits of Eating Pickles

Pickles, especially long term pickles such as naturally fermented sauerkraut aid in the digestion of whole grains. The enzymes and bacteria in naturally fermented vegetables assist in breaking down complex carbohydrates into simple sugars, which will keep our blood sugar level even and may be an important factor in reducing sugar cravings. Also pickles will encourage pancreatic function.

Overeating pickles, however, may actually increase sugar cravings: the substantial quantity of salt present in pickles when eaten in large quantities (more than two tablespoons per day) may create a craving for sweets, sugars, fruits, fruit juices, sodas, liquids in general, alcohol, etc. Salt is a mineral, which has a highly contractive effect on our bodies. To help offset the overabundance of salt and tightening factors in the body, the body naturally tries to make balance by craving sugars, stimulants, alcohol or sodas for example.

Eating pickles on a regular basis will regulate our stomach acids, stomach bacteria, stimulate peristaltic movement in the intestines, as well as replenishing or establishing beneficial bacteria in our digestive tract and other places such as the mucous membranes of the mouth and genital organs. It will prevent unhealthy bacteria from proliferating and becoming active: Umeboshi plum, a traditional Japanese pickled fruit, is known to have antibiotic and antiseptic properties. (as Dr. Kyo Sato of the Hirosaki University proved by showing that nine grams of ume extract could destroy staphyloccus and dysentery bacteria).

Pickling preserves vitamin C in foods, which is a necessary factor in the absorption of iron, and the pickling process strengthens blood and immune function by assisting in splitting organic iron from other nutrients in foods.
The salt factor in pickles helps to keep a slightly alkaline balance of our blood, if eaten in appropriate amounts (approx. one to two tablespoons per day).

# Importance of Microbes in Foods

Molds, yeasts and bacteria are important in food fermentation as well as food spoilage. It is true that molds are involved in the spoilage of many foods, however, some are important in food manufacture especially in fermentation, the preparation of oriental foods, and mold ripened dairy products such as cheese. Various fungi such as the species of Aspergillus, Fusarium, and Penicillium, have been found in foods and are helpful for our bodies, yet some have been implicated in toxin production.

Certain kinds of yeast and koji induce fermentation. Both are in the family of filamentous fungus or molds. Lactic acid fermentation is occurring through certain bacteria, the most known of which is Lactobacillus acidopholus.

Lactobacillus acidophilus occurs naturally in the human and animal gastrointestinal tract, mouth and vagina. The acid produced by *L. acidophilus* in the vagina may help to control a potential overgrowth of the fungus Candida albicans, thus helping to prevent vaginal yeast infections. The same beneficial effect has been observed in cases of oral or gastrointestinal Candidiasis infections.

Some of the important roles played by the lactobacillus acidophilus are suppressing the growth of pathogenic bacteria, boosting the digestive system, helping in the production of vitamins and improving the immune system. There are 400 different types of probiotics and Lactobacillus acidophilus, is one of them. Following is a brief overview of acidophilus benefits.

Natural mold, yeast or lactic acid fermentation is a process of breaking down foods into new components. This new arrangement of components and nutrients is very much guided by active and expanding earth energy. The longer a fermentation process takes, the more it is imbued with the natural rhythms of nature. When consuming long term fermented food items like sauerkraut or miso or kimchi on a regular basis, we can become aware of these inherent cycles of our beautiful planet and we begin to live intuitively more in conjunction with these natural cycles – cycles such as the seasons or the cycles of life and death, etc. Being open to this kind of intuitive understanding gives us access to a wealth of information that is always available, but we have forgotten how to tap into this vast pool of energy and information. Pickles will assist this process.

## Summary of Benefits of Eating Naturally Fermented Foods (uncooked)

- Yeast infections, both vaginal, oral or throughout the digestive system or body as a whole will be reduced and eventually cease when eating good quality long term pickles on a regular basis along with eating a well balanced diet.

- Lactobacillus acidophilus in pickles will boost our immune function by being able to regulate the overgrowth of disease causing bacteria.

- Lactic acid pickles help to produce of a number of chemicals that aid the process of digestion.

- Various digestive problems such as Crohns disease, indigestion, constipation, diarrhea, irritable bowel syndrome, etc, benefit tremendously especially when eating long term pickles (pickled for a minimum of three months).

- It prevents harmful bacteria from producing cancer-causing substances and reduces free radicals, which could potentially damage cells and DNA..

- Lactic acid foods, like sauerkraut absorb cholesterol in the intestine. The effect is lowering the cholesterol levels and boosting the cardio-vascular system.

- The fiber from lactic acid fermented foods help to propel waste out of the digestive system through proper bowel movement, and reduces toxic build up in the body.

- Pickles assist in the manufacture of a number of vitamins in the intestine. Some of them are vitamin K, vitamin B12, Vitamin B1 and folic acid..

- When people suffer from diarrhea or are taking laxatives or antibiotics, beneficial bacteria and micro-organisms are flushed out of the intestines or destroyed, which can weaken their immunity and overall vitality. Naturally long term fermented foods (raw) will remedy this condition if consumed regularly.

# Miso

Miso is a fermented seasoning paste originated in Japan. Most traditional misos are made from soybeans, barley or rice, salt and a fungus called aspergillus oryzae. It contains live enzymes and bacteria that arise through the long fermentation process. These bacteria and enzymes are only present in unpasteurized miso. Fermentation time varies: some misos are fermented or aged several years and others only a few weeks. Miso is low in fat and has absolutely no cholesterol. The bacteria in naturally long term fermented miso have been found to manufacture vitamin B12. Miso, to name some benefits, is used to relieve acid indigestion and other digestive upsets, cardiovascular benefits, anti-cancer benefits. Miso is used to boost the immune function, improve digestive metabolism, and neutralize blood toxins, and thus clear the skin, as well as creating a more alkaline blood condition.

Still another benefit of miso is in its ability to counteract the adverse effects of radiotherapy, antibiotics, chemotherapy and environmental pollution. Dr. Akizuki, who was the director of the department of Internal Medicine at the St. Francis Hospital in Nagasaki after the bombing of Nagasaki in 1945 gave his colleagues a strict diet following the bombing including brown rice, miso, sea vegetables, Hokkaido squash, natural soy sauce and Hokkaido azuki beans. The hospital was located only one mile from the atomic bomb. However, many hospital patients and staff survived acute radiation poisoning sickness without major radiation symptoms, because these foods strengthen the immune function of the body. Stimulated by Dr. Akizuki's experience, Japanese scientists conducted a study of miso in 1972. They discovered a substance called zybicolin in miso, which is produced by the yeasts and fungus during the fermentation process. Zybicolin is able to attract, absorb, and discharge radioactive elements such as strontium. Miso is also able to detoxify the harmful influences of tobacco and traffic pollution.

# Round and Root Vegetables

Round and ground vegetables, such as squash, onion, cabbage, cauliflower, rutabaga, turnips most often become very sweet in flavor when cooked, due to their higher concentration of complex carbohydrates. Generally speaking round vegetables have a stabilizing effect on the body, allowing us to both physically and emotionally stay centered and peaceful.

Root vegetables are more compact and burrow into the solid ground, which attests to their strength and focus. Some root vegetables are more watery like daikon, also called long white radish, while others have a drier texture, like carrots. Many root vegetables store well throughout the winter in a cool room without the need for refrigeration. Eating root vegetables will provide us with strength, focus and endurance.

For more spiritual development of ourselves it is helpful to eat less animal quality foods and more plant based foods. While animal foods are helping us to be very centered in here and now it can also mean that we are being wrapped up in life's immediate drama's constantly without the ability to retain a larger perspective.

However, when choosing to consume more or only plant quality foods, it is important to utilize strengthening cooking methods, especially during the winter time. Too many times young people decide to become vegetarian, but they only consume large quantities of salads, even in the winter, and after a few years of consuming only raw salads, they are surprised to experience various health problems.

Following are some of the more strengthening cooking methods, suitable more for round and root vegetables.

## Nishime Style Cooking

"Ni-" means boiling in Japanese and "-shime" means squeezing. A free translation of this cooking method would be like 'locking in energy cooking style' or 'contracting energy cooking style'.

This dish is traditionally prepared with round and/or root vegetables, which are generally higher in complex carbohydrates than leafy greens and thus have a naturally sweeter flavor, along with providing stabilizing energy and long term sustaining energy.

This cooking method is appropriate all year long, with slight variations: during the warmer season, we cut the vegetables a little smaller and cook this dish more quickly, whereas during the colder months of the year it is helpful to cut the vegetables in large chunks and cook them for a long time until they are sweet and delicious and have a warming effect on the body.

This cooking method is particularly helpful to restore a person's strength and vitality, especially if someone feels physically weakened. If a person has taken large amounts of medication for a long period of time (most medications are classified as having a more yin and expanding/weakening effect in the body) applying this cooking method often will bring the body back to its former resilience more quickly.

Eating this dish creates a particularly peaceful and harmonious body energy: like a pond that during a few days of rain becomes churned up and murky, but once the sunshine returns all of the muck is settling on the bottom of the pond and the water becomes crystal clear and serene again.

Many people in our world are having a condition of hypoglycemia or low blood sugar level. Most people are not diagnosed with this condition, but it is a rampant condition affecting all areas of the populace. Some of the most common symptoms are as follows: sweet cravings or intense hunger pangs, anxiety, sleepiness (often in the early afternoon hours, but may be mid-morning, as well), sweating, weakness, palpitations, confusion when doing routine tasks, some kinds of insomnia among others.

Nishime style cooking counterbalances hypoglycemia and will keep your blood sugar level steady for quite a long time, because of the complex carbohydrates in the sweet vegetables, such as squash, onion and carrots, which are released slowly but steadily into the bloodstream along with fiber, vitamins and minerals and other micro-nutrients. Hypoglycemia also indicates an emotional imbalance: most people that I have seen with this condition are swinging back and forth between moods of elation and hyperactivity on one hand and depression and lethargy on the other. The hyperactivity part lasts as long as the sugar rush from eating sweets, fruits, sodas, café lattes, etc. lasts, and when that wears off, people find themselves in depressed modes of being. This emotional sea-saw dynamic is rooted in an imbalance of the solar plexus chakra (the energy center between the heart and navel). Usually it also goes along with feeling not good enough about oneself, which is played out in either putting oneself down all the time, or doing the opposite: playing out the dynamic of 'I am better than...' to hide the underlying 'less than' feeling. And when this emotional dynamic is played out for many years of one's life, and one cannot trust oneself because one is 'not good enough', then people with this condition begin to become suspicious, critical and untrusting in other people – always suspecting the worst motives in other people's actions.

Physically this imbalance is rooted in a twofold problem: both spleen and pancreas are malfunctioning to a very small or larger degree. The spleen is the intake valve for universal energy, and if it is energetically clogged and weakened, we cannot take in this ever steady-flowing rejuvenating cosmic force and our whole outlook on life becomes stressed and small-minded. The pancreas is also stressed and compressed by other tightening influences like eating too much animal foods, especially chicken and eggs, or losing a loved one, or a stressful job and so on. These influences will reduce the pancreas' ability to release anti-insulin, also called glucagon. Glucagon is produced in the pancreas by so-called alpha cells. Insulin is produced by so-called beta cells. The alpha cells are naturally larger or more expanded than the smaller, more compact beta cells. When we are exposed to a lot of tightening influences in our life, the larger alpha cells are most negatively impacted – they shrink, as opposed to the beta cells, which are less negatively impacted by these tightening influences. Glucagon raises the blood-sugar level, whereas insulin lowers it. When we eat something sweet to relax the tension we feel in our bodies, insulin is being released because the insulin producing cells are still functioning properly. The blood sugar level drops because insulin is released. Often, the blood sugar level drops too low, because the glucagon releasing cells are overly compressed and are not releasing glucagon to the degree that is necessary to balance out the blood sugar level. This results in low blood sugar level, which in turn will make us crave more sweets or stimulants, again, to keep or get going. When we continue this pattern of eating for many years, we often are prone to diabetes later on in life.

Nishime style cooking will help to bring our organs back to proper functioning. Selecting more round vegetables, like onions and squash and rutabaga, will produce a more relaxing effect, counterbalancing hypoglycemia. Selecting more root vegetables like carrots, burdock, parsnips or daikon, for example, will be more helpful for stronger warming energy, strengthening the digestive function, alleviating skin problems and counterbalancing the weakening side effects of most medications.

This is a long cooking vegetable dish. People often ask how this cooking method can be beneficial, when according to their understanding many nutrients will be lost by cooking this dish so long. Here is the answer: If you are eating leafy greens 2 or 3 times per day, using raw vegetables or short cooking methods like pressed salad, quick blanching, quick steaming or quick sauté, then you are not relying on the heat sensitive nutrients in this dish. The Vitamin B-complex nutrients are generally not heat sensitive and will not be lost. Most of the root and round vegetables are not high in vitamin C content, which is heat sensitive. The effect of this dish is slightly or strongly warming, depending on the length of cooking time. Imagine eating only raw cucumbers in the winter time, just the thought of it can make you feel cold – unless you have eaten too much animal food, which can produce and overheating effect in the body and thus eating cucumbers in the winter for a person with a an overheated body that may feel good.

Nishime feels nourishing and warming particularly during the colder months of the year.

Generally speaking it is important to consume some stabilizing or slightly warming foods to retain our body heat and keep our internal energy source going and some neutral or slightly cooling foods. Depending on the season, we may select more of one category or another.

Another important factor is actually the size of a pot: Select a pot for this dish or any dish for that matter, that is appropriate for the amount of vegetables or ingredients that will be placed into the pot. If the pot is mostly empty, then the taste will be mostly that of a vacuum, if the pot on the other hand is 2/3 or ¾ full, the dish will taste stronger and more delicious. Other factors are important for taste as well, such as the amount of oil and salt or season agents added to the food.

When cooking in stainless steel or copper pots, it is important not to stir with metal utensils in the pot when possible, because the electromagnetic charge between two metal objects rubbing against each other (when stirring with a metal spoon in a metal pot, for example) influences the taste of the food in a disadvantageous way.

# Kinpira Style Cooking

Kinpira is a dish that requires a little more effort in terms of preparation, and more care during the cooking process than nishime. The result is well worth it, both taste-wise and in regards to the energy it produces in the body. Most often we use a combination of two or more root vegetables like carrots and burdock in equal amounts. Roots have a more strengthening, focusing energy, as they are highly charged by heaven's downward force, growing down into the earth. This cooking method is used often especially in cases of feeling tired or exhausted, experiencing indigestion, anemia, skin diseases and other excessively yin conditions like breast cancer, chronic constipation and many more. While the actual cooking time is not as long as the nishime style cooking, then energy of this dish is more like a concentrated shot of energy.

Any energy we put into a dish, will return to us 100-fold when eating the dish. First we use a lot of energy to cut all the vegetables into thin matchstick slices.

Then we begin the actual cooking process by sautéing one of the root vegetables. When using burdock and carrot, we sauté the burdock in a skillet first separately. This part of the cooking method is more activating. Next we layer the second vegetable on top of the first and adding enough water to only cover the burdock or the bottom layer of vegetables.

Then we bring the liquid to a boil, cover the skillet and let the vegetables cook over a low flame for 10 – 20 minutes or until the vegetables are almost completely soft. This part of the cooking process is more peaceful, and quieting. After the quiet cooking time we add soy sauce, and mix the vegetables, turn the flame up high for a moment to evaporate any left over liquid and drive the flavor back into the vegetables.  Finally, remove from the heat and serve hot or warm. This last part of the cooking method is more activating, and strengthening, again.

You may now understand the process of this cooking method and looking at the energetic pattern when preparing this dish moving from high energy, to low energy and finally high energy again. This dish is quite a bit more activating and giving us a quick injection of energy that is highly focusing.

Please be aware that organically or naturally grown vegetables have a much higher nutrient content than their conventionally grown counterparts. If you buy produce from your local farmer, the foods are picked ripe and reaching your dinner table in prime condition, versus produce that has been picked before it ripens and is transported thousands of miles to reach your grocery store. Sometimes local farmers do not have the organic label certificate – a process that is lengthy and expensive – but still their produce is grown by the same natural methods. The quality and benefit may be even greater than organic labeled vegetables imported from other regions of the country or the world. When foods are grown and harvested in a local environment they are more strengthening for a person living in that area, because the vegetables are grown in local soil and exposed to the local celestial bodies, thus providing the person with nutrients and energy information particularly suitable for her or his area.

If you wish to reach for an even more beneficial effect on the body and mind: grow your own vegetables in a very specific way: Take some seeds of each vegetable and place them under your tongue for nine minutes. This will imbue the seeds with your DNA. Next remove the seeds from your mouth and place them into your hands, preferably standing barefoot on the soil you are going to grow the vegetables in. Lift your hands with the seeds up to the heavens and ask for the grace of the divine celestial bodies and energies to assist in the process of the growth of these special vegetables. Then you gently blow on the seeds in your hands to provide even more specific information about yourself to the vegetables from your breath. Afterwards create little holes in the soil for the seeds to be placed into and spit into the hole before you insert the seed and cover it with soil. Do not water the seeds right away - instead wait 1 – 3 days before watering. This allows each seed to fully grasp the information it is surrounded by.

Vegetables, and plants in general, are strongly service oriented. When we engage a seed to grow specifically for us, this seed will do it's utmost to provide us with nutrients and energy (within its range of capabilities) that is best for our health, wellbeing and spiritual growth. If a plant senses an imbalance or illness, it will grow with the intent to regain this person's health. Perhaps you don't have a garden or don't have time for a garden, you can grow a few herbs this way on a windowsill. It will have a very beneficial effect. The exchange between plants and humans is much greater than we currently are aware of in our age of intellectual knowledge and science. We cannot ever truly understand nature's glorious inner complexities and magical interconnectedness with everything else living on this planet by killing it first and then separating its individual components. However, we can slowly become aware of the intricate connections by truly experiencing them and hearing nature's song without and within us.

# Examining Representatives of each of the Vegetable Categories:

I would like to examine one representative of each of the three vegetable categories (leafy greens, round vegetables and root vegetables) further.

**Leafy Greens: Kale**
**Round Vegetables: Cabbage**
**Root Vegetables: Burdock**

# Kale

Many of you may be familiar with kale. I have often seen it in stores as decoration in the deli sections – as kale is hardy and won't wilt quickly. There are many different varieties of kale, some curly, some open, some more dark green, some light green or whitish and some purple/bluish in color. The kale plant is large when fully matured. The sometimes expansive leaves are reaching out in all directions around the central stem and they love cool or cold weather. Traditionally kale leaves were harvested after the first frost, to bring out a sweeter, richer flavor. Summer kale is somewhat more bitter in taste, but delicious nonetheless. Looking at the structure of how kale grows, we can gather that the energetic effect of ingesting kale is more opening, relaxing, and activating, yet keeping our core strong.

Should you deem yourself more introverted and would like to socialize more easily, I would suggest eating foods like kale and other leafy greens whose leaves stretch out like antennae in all directions for making contact and connection. Emphasis on leafy greens such as kale is also helpful when our energetic center seems too low in the body. For example, when we feel heavy or when compact and dense growths, such as fibroids, cysts or tumors (especially in the lower part of the body) are developing, emphasis on consuming larger amounts of leafy greens rather than round or root vegetables will be helpful.

Kale is a high fiber content food, which helps to propel waste and toxins out of our digestive system through bowel movement and is thus very cleansing for our bodies. Like other cruciferous vegetables such as broccoli, brussel sprouts or cabbage, kale contains a substance called glucoraphanin. When cutting or chewing kale this substance transforms into sulforaphane under the influence of the enzyme myrosinase. Sulforaphane is known for its anticancerous, antidiabetic and antimicrobial properties. This substance inspires the liver to create special enzymes, which help in eliminating chemicals that can cause or contribute to cancer growth.

Kale furthermore contains large amounts of flavonoids. These substances are known for their anti-allergic, anti-inflammatory, anti-microbial, anti-cancer, strengthening cardio-vascular system and antioxidant activity. The antioxidant abilities of flavonoids may be stronger than those of Vitamin C and E.

Certain antioxidants available in kale and a substance called indole-3-carbinol disable free radicals, so that they can't damage DNA, fat containing molecules or cell membranes.

Kale contains quite a bit of Vitamin C – 1 cup of fresh kale, chopped, contains more than an average person's daily needs of vitamin C. And vitamin C is a well known booster for our immune function.

The complex plant nutrients in kale allow our bodies to produce enzymes that are important in the detoxification process. This helps our bodies to cleanse and remove toxins not only from our intestines, but the detoxification properties of kale benefit the skin, the lungs, the reproductive organs, and the liver, as well. The bitter components in kale help the liver to produce bile, which in turn helps our digestive function.

Kale contains very high amounts of Vitamin A and (Pro-Vitamin A such as) carotenoids, which are substances that work to protect our eyes from damage when exposed to ultraviolet light.

Of course kale is also packed with chlorophyll – the green pigment in plants, which help in our bodies to pick up toxins such as heavy metals, pesticides, herbicides and other toxins to be eliminated through bowel movement.

Also, kale is stuffed with a wealth of other nutrients: Vitamin E, Vitamin B6, Vitamin K, Folate, Calcium, Potassium, Manganese, Iron and Zinc.

Bananas are touted for their potassium rich content. However not only bananas are good sources for potassium, in fact kale is a very good source of potassium, without the cooling and weakening effects of eating bananas in a cold climate during the winter.

When it comes to calcium and iron, kale is a very important player, as well, because the vitamin C content in kale assists in the absorption of calcium and iron.

Also, vitamin A and zinc work together in kale to fight toxins and help your immune system to work better. They assist the immune system in creating white blood cells. This is significant in the prevention of infections, and viruses.

Kale provides a great dose of vitamin K, to prevent heavy bleeding (in case of heavy menstrual bleeding for example) and vitamin K is important for bone metabolism. Manganese, similarly, is important for the formation of strong bones, and also building or maintaining a healthy nervous system and helping thyroid function.

As you can see, Kale is packed with health benefits. You may wish to look at other leafy greens in depth as well, to find out about their wealth of life-giving qualities. Or simply eat them and find out which ones you like best, because in most cases our bodies tell us by 'like' or 'dislike' which leafy greens, or any vegetables for that matter, are most appropriate and suitable for retaining our health and vibrancy or the regaining thereof through our resilient natures.

# Cabbage

I believe everybody is familiar with regular, green or red cabbage. Cabbage is one of my favorite vegetables all year round – it is sturdy, abundant, easy to grow or inexpensive to buy and stores well.

As opposed to kale, which is extending and expanding in all directions, cabbage is more conservative and closed in on itself. Thus the energy of cabbage is more centering and stabilizing. In case of over-activity in our body, such as inflammation, cabbage is the perfect food choice or it may be applied as an external plaster to counterbalance such a condition.

If you have ever seen cabbages grow in a garden or on a farm you can sense their unshakable beingness. They are what they are, they are content and happy within themselves and nothing can shake them out of their peaceful, yet cheery quality of life. Thus, when we feel emotionally unstable and challenged, cabbage is happy to imbue us with its soothing and stable nature, so that we may return to our cheery, happy and content selves.

Cabbage is an excellent source of vitamin C, also a good source of Thiamin, vitamin B6, Folate, Calcium, Potassium, Iron, Magnesium and Manganese.

Cabbage is free of cholesterol, but high in fiber, which will help in to propel waste and toxins out of our digestive system through bowel movement. It is very cleansing for our bodies. The fiber-related compounds in cabbage and other cruciferous vegetables bind with bile acids in the digestive tract and this allows the bile acids to be excreted. For proper digestion, the liver needs to replace the depleted supply of bile acids by drawing upon our existing quantity of cholesterol in the body, resulting in lowering our cholesterol level. This benefit is not decreased by lightly cooking cabbage, in fact studies have shown that the cholesterol-lowering ability of cabbage improves drastically when steamed[11]. Lowering our cholesterol levels is well known for positively impacting our cardio-vascular system.

The antioxidant power of green and red cabbage is well known, especially due to vitamin A and its pro-vitamins, the carotenoids, as well as a group of substances called polyphenols. What do antioxidants do? They have the power to prevent a chain reaction from happening within cells, by removing free radicals to prevent the damage or death of a cell. Damaged cells can more easily be susceptible to cancerous activity; hence antioxidants play a role in

---

[11] Kahlon TS, Chiu MC, Chapman MH. Steam cooking significantly improves in vitro bile acid binding of collard greens, kale, mustard greens, broccoli, green bell pepper, and cabbage. 2008 Jun;28(6):351-7. 2008.

cancer prevention and shrinkage of existing cancer. Anthocyanin, a polyphenyl occurring in red cabbage, is also known to be strongly anti-inflammatory.

Laboratory-based information has also provided evidence for other potential health effects such as delaying or blocking aging and neurological diseases, diabetes, bacterial infections and fibrocystic disease.

It also contains significant amounts of glutamin, which is an amino acid that is credited with anti-inflammatory properties.

The best anti-cancer and health benefits in cabbage, however, are found in a phytonutrient category called glucosinolates. These substances change into isothiocyanate compounds when cabbage is chewed or cut via a specific plant enzyme (myrosinase) present in the cabbage. This enzyme is only activated when the leaves are injured such as through chewing or cutting. Glucosinolates offer a protection from a variety of cancers such as bladder cancer, breast cancer, colon cancer.

Like kale, cabbage is also a good source of flavonoids. These substances are known for their anti-allergic, anti-inflammatory, anti-microbial, anti-cancer, strengthening cardio-vascular system and antioxidant activity. The antioxidant abilities of flavonoids and a substance called indole-3-carbinol disable free radicals, so that they can't damage fat containing molecules, cell membranes or DNA and in fact they are boosting DNA repair and blocking the growth of cancer cells.

Fresh cabbage juice is known to have a rapid improvement on the healing of peptic ulcers[12]. As more studies about this powerful food are undertaken, it becomes clear that cabbage contains a variety of substances that are protecting and benefitting our stomach and intestinal linings. Heliobacter pylori, which is a naturally occurring bacteria in the stomach, can under certain conditions overpopulate and create unwanted symptoms such as duodenal ulcers or even stomach cancer. Cabbage can be of assistance in the regulation of the bacterial population.

While I am not about to list all of the wonderful substances in cabbage, this might give you a good idea, but even better: please include cabbage in your diet on a regular bases, at least 3 – 5 times per week!

## Burdock Root

Burdock is a long, relatively thin, brown skinned root. Some of my students called it a short walking stick – and rightly so: it can look like a walking stick. It is a somewhat dry root, perhaps like parsnip. The inside color of the root is cream colored. Most people are familiar with the sticky burrs, which the burdock plant produces to hold and carry its seed.

---

[12] Calif. Med. 1949 January; 70(1): 10 – 15; Garnett Cheney; Rapid Healing of Peptic Ulcers in Patients Receiving Fresh Cabbage Juice; PMCID: PMC1643665

The burrs are sticking easily to clothing, hair and really anything – natures true inspiration for Velcro. Burdock is a two year plant: the first year it develops a good root and leaves and in the second year all the energy stored in the root gets projected upward into the plant so that it will produce the seeds (located within the burrs).

Burdock has been long touted as a blood purifier by various eastern and western traditional cultures – it is known to remove toxins that can build up in our blood. Also burdock root has a diuretic effect and can relieve swelling in ankles and soothe aching joints, because it helps to eradicate uric acid, which can build up in joints and cause pain.

Burdock grows easily in cooler climates, it doesn't need any special care while growing at all, and in fact is often considered an obnoxious weed. However, the strength that is carried within this brown root can be best described through the words 'resilient' 'sturdy' and even 'tough'.

Even though the root looks dark brown, I would still consider this plant as more feminine in nature than kale or cabbage. I would liken it perhaps to a female sage, utterly unique, independent, wild, and yet wise. She knows about slow, persistent growth, and that certain stages of development will take time to mature. A strong being and a strong ally.

Chlorogenic acid, one of burdock's active ingredients, is an antioxidant, which has many benefits: it slows the release of glucose into the bloodstream after a meal, it acts as an inhibitor of tumor promoting activity, it is thought to contribute to the prevention of Type 2 Diabetes and cardiovascular disease, as well as having antiviral, antibacterial and antifungal properties.

Inulin is another wonderful ingredient in burdock, which is known as a sugar, that has minimal impact on the blood sugar level and doesn't raise the triglyceride level thus making it a suitable vegetable for diabetics and other blood sugar related diseases.

Another substance found in burdock are lactones - these help the prevention of biofilms in the body, which in turn prevents detrimental microbes from hiding in one's body.

Even though burdock is a relatively dry root, it does contain a gluey substance, called mucilage. This substance is medicinally used to alleviate inflammatory processes of any of the mucous membranes of the body, by covering them and preventing irritation of the nerve endings.

Considering that we as humans experience everything through our senses, we believe that this universe is quite physical and dense in some areas and empty in others. However, physics tells us that what we are experiencing with our senses is fooling us, because even each atom is not quite physical at all.

The particles of which an atom is made up of are a combination of wave and particle and the space in-between the nucleus of a an atom and its electrons is comparatively as void as the space between the stars in the galaxies. So, our bodies are a large void of space with some electrical discharge and information distribution. Burdock contains polyacetylene, which is an organic compound that is a highly conducive conductor for electricity. In order to charge ourselves up more and allow for a better electrical body system, burdock will be a wonderful addition to anyone's diet.

Taraxosterol is another active ingredient found in burdock, which has anti-tumor properties, along with anti-inflammatory, cholesterol-lowering, anti-microbial, anti-bacterial and anti-fungal effects.

Also the usual housekeeping: burdock is very high in fiber, and a good source of vitamin B6, magnesium, potassium and manganese.

When someone is suffering from skin trouble like acne, eczema or psoriasis, burdock will be a powerful ally, because it provides natural compounds to heal the skin (also the anti-inflammatory properties are important), and more importantly it will re-direct excess and toxic waste away from the surface of the body to be discharged through the regular channels of bowel movement and urination. Burdock's energy is strongly downward and inward directed, so will counterbalance excess that may have been rising to the surface of the body and higher up in the body — like pimples on the face.

# Vegetable Recipes

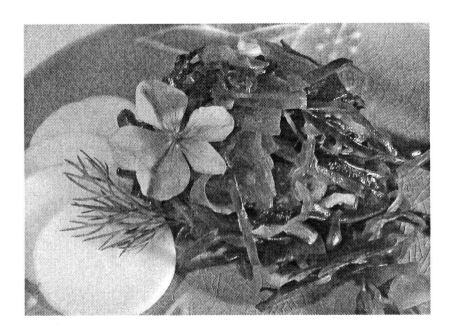

Red Cabbage – Sweet and Sour, German Style, see
page 125

# Kinpira Soup

3 tablespoons of burdock root, carrot, lotus root
(dried or fresh), onion and sweet winter squash
(butternut, kabocha, buttercup, red kuri)
1 dried shiitake mushroom, soaked and minced
sesame oil
sea salt
water
chickpea miso (or other short term fermented miso)
2 year fermented barley miso
minced scallion or parsley for garnish

Mince burdock, carrot and lotus root. Lightly brush
the bottom of the soup pot with sesame oil and heat
on a medium flame. When oil is hot, saute the
burdock for 2 - 3 minutes. Layer the shiitake, carrot
and lotus root on top of burdock. Cover all vegetables
with water, gently bring to a boil with a pinch of salt,
and lower the flame - simmer for 10 to 20 minutes.
You may need to add water from time to time to
prevent complete evaporation and burning of the
vegetables. Add minced onion and sweet winter
squash next. Add enough water to cover all
vegetables, and simmer until all the vegetables are
tender – approximately 20 – 30 minutes. Mix the two
kinds of miso in a small bowl and dilute with some
soup broth. Slowly add diluted miso to soup for a
mild (not salty) flavor. Simmer another 2 - 3 minutes.
This stew should be thick, like a hearty stew. Garnish
with scallions or parsley.

# Kinpira

burdock
carrot
sesame oil
soy sauce or tamari
toasted, crushed sesame seeds (optional)
fresh squeezed ginger juice

Cut equal amounts of burdock and carrots (if burdock is not available, you may use lotus root, parsnips, rutabaga or onions) into matchsticks or very small pieces.
Lightly brush a skillet with oil. When the oil is hot, sauté the burdock matchsticks for several minutes in a skillet or frying pan. Then layer the carrot matchsticks on top of the burdock. Next add enough water to barely cover the burdock, not the carrots. Place the lid on the skillet. Cook until the vegetables are 80 % done. This may take 10 – 20 minutes or longer. Towards the end of cooking time add a small amount of soy sauce or tamari and simmer for at least another five minutes. Leave the skilled un-covered. Cook until all water has evaporated. Optional: Add a few drops of freshly squeezed ginger juice at the end of cooking and/or a small amount of toasted, crushed sesame seeds.

# Nishime Style Cooking
# Onion Nishime – Heart Muscle Restorative

5 medium sized onions, cut into large chunks or wedges
1 inch piece of kombu, soaked
2 minced umbeshi plums or sea salt
water
minced parsley

Use a heavy pot with a heavy lid – when using a light weight pot you may have to add water during the cooking process to prevent burning.
Place the kombu in the pot first, then add the onion chunks and sprinkle the minced umeboshi plums or sea salt on top. Finally add a small amount of water – enough to cover the bottom of the pot by ¼ inch. Cover the pot and bring to a boil. Lower the flame and simmer one to two hours. Remove the lid, turn off the flame, and let the vegetables sit for a few minutes. Serve any remaining liquid along with the vegetables or thicken the liquid with kuzu as a glaze over the onions. Garnish with parsley.

Variations:
- Add other vegetables cut into large chunks and cook them slowly over a long time over low heat. This allows the ingredients to be cooked in their own juices, almost exclusively.

- Use soy sauce for seasoning towards the end of cooking (simmer it for the last 5 minutes of cooking) instead of using sea salt or umeboshi plum.
- Vegetable combination suggestions:

Carrot, onions, parsnip, burdock, cabbage, shiitake and kombu

Carrot, burdock, onions, squash, celery and kombu

Squash, onion, daikon, rutabaga and kombu

Daikon, lotus root, carrot, burdock and kombu,

Daikon, shiitake and kombu,

# Steamed Leafy Greens

(Kale, collards, watercress, chinese cabbage, bok choy, radish tops, carrot tops, turnip tops, mustard greens, etc.)

Wash and slice your choice of green, leafy vegetable(s). Place approximately 1 inch of water into a sauce pan with a stainless steel or bamboo steamer inset and bring the water to a boil. Next, place a small amount of your vegetables into the steamer - a large amount of vegetables is generally not cooking evenly and resulting in partly overcooked vegetables. Cover (optional) and steam for 1 – 3 minutes, depending on the texture of the vegetable. Remove and transfer quickly to a serving dish, to prevent overcooking. Then proceed in the same manner with the remaining vegetables.

Allow the bright green color and crispness of the vegetabales to be your guide – bright green indicates the presence of vitamin C, whereas grey or dull green suggests that vitamin C has been destroyed through the prolonged cooking process.

## Blanched Vegetables

Bring several inches of water to a boil in a pot with a pinch of sea salt.  Drop in a small amount of vegetables and boil for 10 seconds up to 2 minutes. Remove the vegetables quickly and place them in a strainer to drain.

This kind of cooking method may be used with one kind of vegetable or several vegetables. It is more often used with leafy greens or leafy greens in combination with root or round vegetables. When preparing a mixed blanched vegetable salad, cook each vegetable separately, in the same boiling water.

For example:
carrots, cut into matchsticks
daikon, sliced into matchsticks
watercress, sliced into one inch slices
arugual, sliced into one inch slices

Blanche these vegetables, separately, one at a time, in the same boiling water, beginning with the carrot matchsticks, then the daikon matchsticks, then watercress, and finally arugula. Squeeze out excessive liquid out of greens at the end. Mix all vegetables or arrange them on a serving platter and serve as is or with a dressing.

In order to retain distinctive cooking flavors, begin by blanching the mildest tasting vegetables first and proceed towards the stronger flavored vegetables.

When cooking greens with this method, remove the leafy greens from the boiling water before the color has dulled. A vibrant green color is an indicator that vitamin C is still intact.

Small or fine slicing is important for this cooking method, as it is a short cooking method. Large chunks of vegetables generally take longer to cook.

Blanched vegetables may be served as is or with a dressing or condiment of your choice.

# Sesame – Miso – Dressing

Sort, wash and roast and grind sesame seeds. Mix ground sesame seeds with a miso of your choice (light colored miso has a milder taste in most cases) and dilute to desired consistency with left over liquid from the blanching process. Add a small amount of grated onion, if desired. Pour over blanched vegetables and serve.

# Blanched Watercress with Tangerine Dressing

1 bunch watercress
1 small head of endive for garnish
water for blanching
dressing: fresh pressed tangerine juice or fresh
pressed orange juice (3-4 tangerines or oranges)
1 – 2 teaspoons Dijon mustard or to taste
1 – 2 teaspoons fresh pressed ginger juice or to taste

Blanche watercress. Arrange on serving platter.

Squeeze orange or tangerine juice into a bowl. Whisk juice, mustard and ginger until evenly mixed. Arrange the raw endive in a circular pattern on a serving platter, then fill each endive leaf with a small amount of blanched watercress. Drizzle dressing over the blanched watercress and endive. Serve.

# Quickly Sautéed Vegetables

Leafy greens, sliced and finely sliced root or round vegetables as well as sprouts or corn may be sautéed, by themselves or in various combinations.
Heat a small amount of oil or water in a skillet to sauté the vegetables briefly. Gently stir the vegetables with a wooden utensil. Sprinkle with a little sea salt, soy sauce, or tamari and simmer a few minutes longer, adding water when necessary to prevent burning.

When I cook leafy greens this way, I most often choose a dark green variety along with a light green variety for contrast of color and flavor. Root or round vegetables such as carrots and onions are wonderful additions to this dish, but need to be cooked just a little longer than leafy greens.

1 cup cabbage, finely sliced
1 cup onion or leek, finely sliced
1 cup kale, sliced finely or torn into small pieces
olive or sesame oil
sea salt
water as needed

Heat a small amount of oil in a skillet and begin by sautéing the onions (or leeks). When the onions have become glassy, add a few pinches of salt as well as the cabbage. Continue sautéing the vegetables until the cabbage has softened a bit, as well. If a little water is needed during the cooking process to prevent burning, add a few tablespoons of water to the skillet, as needed. Finally add the kale and sauté all the ingredients for another minute or two, until the kale has become tender, but not overcooked.
Transfer to a serving platter and serve immediately.

# Red Radish and Tops

a small bunch of red radishes and tops
water
sea salt or ume vinegar or soy sauce

Slice the red radishes into quarters or thin slices, depending on their size and place them into a skillet with a small amount of water and a pinch or sea salt. Cover the skillet and cook approximately two to three minutes with a few drops of ume vinegar or sea salt. Meanwhile slice the tops finely. Place the cut leaves on top of the roots, then simmer for one or two minutes longer.

Variation: Daikon and Daikon Leaves or Dandelion Roots and Dandelion Tops or Carrots and Tops – as these vegetables are little bit harder than red radishes the cooking time will be slightly longer.

.

# Pressed Salad # 1

3 – 4 chinese cabbage or napa leaves, finely chopped
a three inch piece of fresh lotus root, cut into thin half rounds
½ apple, cut into thin slices
a two inch piece of wakame, soaked and sliced finely
1 scallion, finely sliced
umeboshi vinegar to taste (approximately 2 teaspoons of umeboshi vinegar per cup of sliced vegetables)
3 – 5 tablespoons of roasted walnuts for garnish

In a bowl, mix all the vegetables, sea vegetable and apple. Add umeboshi vinegar to create a slightly salty flavor. Transfer into a salad press and press for 45 minutes or until the liquid level rises above the vegetable level. Discard excess liquid and serve topped with roasted walnuts.

# Pressed Salad # 2

½ cup cucumber, washed and sliced into thin slices
½ cup red radishes, washed and finely sliced
½ cup carrot, washed and grated
1 ½ cups iceberg lettuce, sliced into large chunks
sea salt to taste (approximately ½ teaspoon per cup of sliced vegetables, more if using very hard vegetables)

In a bowl mix the washed and sliced vegetables with the sea salt. Transfer the vegetable mixture into a salad press or you may wish to place the vegetables into a straight edged container (such as a crock pot), placing a flat plate that fits inside the container on top of the vegetables. Then add a weight on top of the plate.

Let the vegetables sit between 10 to 15 minutes (or 30 to 60 minutes if cabbage is used) until the water is drawn out of the vegetables.

Discard the water before serving. If desired add a few drops of lemon juice before serving. If the vegetables are too salty, rinse the vegetables with fresh water.

# Kim Chee

½ cup Chinese cabbage or napa, finely sliced
½ cup cabbage, shredded
1/8 cup leeks, finely sliced
1 – 2 scallions, finely sliced
¼ cup carrots, cut into matchsticks
¼ cup daikon, cut into matchsticks
3 – 4 tablespoons of red pepper, sliced into small cubes or minced
1 – 2 teaspoons ginger, sliced into paper thin matchsticks
1 - 2 cloves garlic, minced
2 – 3 cups water
2 – 4 teaspoons of sea salt

Boil the water with the sea salt. Let cool in a glass or pickling jar.

Place finely cut vegetables into the brine. All the vegetables should be immersed in the salt water. Cover the jar with cheesecloth and let sit in a shady, cool place for 24 hours.

Then remove the cheesecloth, replace it with the lid of the jar and place it into the refrigerator. Only remove the amount of vegetables from the brine you are going to serve with a meal. All the other vegetables can remain in the brine in the refrigerator for approximately one week to 10 days.

# Whole Umeboshi Pickles

2-3 umeboshi plums, pit removed and minced
1 cup water
½ c small cauliflower florets
½ cup carrots, sliced finely
½ cup snap peas, cut into small strips
(finely sliced rutabaga is very nice, but any round or
root vegetables of your choice can be delicious)

Place the minced umeboshi plums into a jar with the
water. Close the jar with the lid and shake the jar
until the plums mix well with the water. Let this
mixture sit for 1 day before inserting any vegetables.

After inserting the vegetables, let it ferment for a
minimum of 3 days, before starting to eat this pickle.

# Shiitake-Onion Pickles, Sweet and Sour

1 cup onions, finely sliced into thin half moons
4 – 5 dried shiitake mushrooms, soaked and sliced
thinly
1/8 cup soy sauce or tamari
1 – 2 teaspoons rice vinegar
3 – 5 tablespoons rice syrup
½ cup water

Blanche the onion half moon pieces for 20 – 30
seconds. Cook the sliced shiitake in their soaking

water for approximately 5 – 10 minutes or until soft. Mix soy sauce and water in a bowl in a ratio of one part soy sauce to three parts of water and add a small amount of rice vinegar and rice syrup to taste. Place the blanched onion slices and cooked shiitake into a glass jar or pickling crock. Pour the brine mixture over the vegetables, completely covering the vegetables. Cover the jar or crock with cheesecloth and let sit in a shady, cool place for 24 hours. After 24 hours remove the cheesecloth, replace it with the lid of the jar and place it into the refrigerator. Only remove the amount of vegetables that you are going to serve right away. All the other vegetables can remain in the brine in the refrigerator for approximately 4 to 10 days.

## Broccoli Stem Shoyu Pickles

1 cup matchstick cut broccoli stems
¼ - 1/3 cup shoyu
¾ cup water

Place all ingredients into a glass jar and cover the jar with cheesecloth. Let is sit at room temperature for 24 hours. After the 24 hours, remove the cheesecloth. Cover the jar with the original screw lid and place into the refrigerator. This pickle will last a minimum of 3 days, but often as long as 2 weeks.

# Spicy Carrot-Squash Soup

2 cups carrots, cut into chunks
2 cups hard winter squash, such as buttercup,
butternut or kabocha, cubed
water
sea salt
1 – 3 teaspoons ginger juice
parsley and/or nori for garnish

If using a tough skinned squash or a green skinned squash, remove the skin (save the skin as it can be cut into small strips and cooked into soups and sautés).

Place the carrot chunks and squash cubes into a soup pot and barely cover with water. Add a pinch of sea salt and bring to a boil. Reduce the flame to low and cover the soup pot. Simmer for 15 to 20 minutes or until all of the vegetables are soft.

Next puree the carrot and squash chunks in a hand food mill or blender and return the pureed liquid to the pot. Add sea salt to taste and cook for another 7 to 10 minutes.

Grate enough ginger so that you can squeeze 1 – 3 teaspoons of ginger juice or to taste and add to the soup towards the end. Garnish with parsley and/or nori strips.

# Red Cabbage – Sweet and Sour, German Style

1 medium sized red cabbage, sliced thinly
2 onions, sliced into thin half moons
2 apples, peeled, cored and sliced into thin slices
1 – 2 tablespoons sesame oil
1 teaspoon sea salt or to taste
½ cup water
1 tablespoon umeboshi vinegar or to taste
3 – 4 bayleaves, optional
½ cup rice syrup

Place the oil into a sauce pan and slowly heat it up. Test heat of the oil with one slice of onion. If the onion slice is sizzling, add the rest of the onions and sauté until they become glassy. Add the thinly sliced apples next, then the red cabbage, the salt and tuck the bayleaves in at the side of the pot. Add water to keep the ingredients from burning in the beginning. Cover and bring to a boil, then turn the heat down low. Simmer for approximately 1 hour. Season with umeboshi vinegar to taste and add rice syrup. Simmer a little longer until all the tastes are mingled and the cabbage is very soft. Serve hot or warm.

# Dried Cranberry Pine Nut Topping over Nishime Style

1 cup dried, minced dried cranberries (fruit juice sweetened cranberries or raisins)
1/3 cup water
½ cup finely sliced oil-cured black olives
2 tablespoons olive oil
1tablespoon balsamic vinegar
1 ½ teaspoons capers, minced
1 ½ teaspoons parsley, minced
½ cup lightly roasted pine nuts (or walnuts, sliced into small pieces)
nishime style cooked vegetables (see page 113)
pinch of sea salt

Bring the cranberries, pinch of sea salt and the water to a boil in a skillet, simmer until the cranberries are soft and the water has evaporated. Add olive oil during the last 2 minutes of cooking. Transfer to a mixing bowl and stir in olives, vinegar, capers and parsley. Set aside. Cook vegetables nishime style until they are soft (daikon, onions, rutabaga, squash, carrots, sweet potato, leek, celery, burdock, cauliflower). Mix pine nuts into topping and gently fold topping into vegetables or serve a small amount of the mixture on top of each individual serving. Serve warm or room temperature.

# Grated Daikon Soup with Mochi

2 cups daikon, washed and finely grated
4 - 5 cups water, including kombu and shiitake
soaking water
2 - 3 inch strip of dry kombu, soaked
4 - 5 dried shiitake, soaked, stems removed and diced
2 - 4 teaspoons of salt or to taste
¼ cup scallions, finely sliced
4 - 5 pieces of mochi, pan fried

Place the water, kombu and shiitake in a pot. Cover and bring to a boil. Reduce the flame to medium and simmer for 5 to 10 minutes.

Remove the kombu and set aside for use in other dishes. Cover and simmer shiitake for another 5 minutes. Add the daikon and sea salt. Cover and simmer over a low flame for another 10 minutes.

Place pan fried mochi in serving bowls, then ladle the soup into the bowls and garnish with sliced scallions.

# Carrot Dill Soup

2 - 3 tablespoons olive oil
1 onion, diced finely
1 lb carrots, cleaned and diced
1 rib celery, leaves included, diced
2 - 3 cups of water or vegetable stock
1/8 cup dill, minced
1 - 2 teaspoons salt or to taste
1/8 teaspoon pepper
minced dill or parsley for garnish

Saute onions in the olive oil first. Then add celery and carrots and saute a moment longer. Next add water or vegetable stock and the remaining ingredients and simmer for approximately 40 minutes. Puree the soup with a blender and serve with dill or other parsley for garnish.

# Sea Vegetables

Growing up by the sea shore, the Baltic Sea and the North Sea, I was familiar with sea vegetables from an early age, as we frequently found them washed ashore. When the tide is out and you walk out onto the dry seabed, you can see various sea vegetables growing on the rocks.

At that time in my life we would use the sea vegetables to grace our sand castles, or we would find them in sea food markets as decoration, but generally we were not used to eating them, unless on rare occasions.

Many years have passed since then, and my son and I are very fond of eating sea vegetables, also called seaweeds.

While sea vegetables contain quite a wide variety of nutrients, such as vitamins A, B complex, C, D, E, and K, their main strength lies in minerals. Sea vegetables are made up of 7-38% of their dry weight in minerals, such as calcium, magnesium, sodium, potassium, iodine, phosphorus, iron, zinc, manganese, vanadium, titanium, copper, cobalt, magnetite, selenium and molybdenum. This wide variety of minerals is generally not available in other categories of plant foods.

Sea vegetables are flexible plants that sway with the ocean's currents and movements. When we look at other sources of minerals, such as salt (especially rock salt, like Himalaya salt) or coral, these sources are crystallized and hard – less flexible. Sea vegetables on the other hand when taken directly from the ocean or rehydrated are pliable and able to adjust to various external conditions with ease without disintegrating. Thus, the effect of eating these flexible vegetables from the sea is strengthening as well as providing us with a similar kind of flexible nature for both our physical and mental/emotional bodies.
And yet: eating sea vegetables to change stubborn character traits without an intense desire and a readiness for a change of character, will not change anyone's characteristics.

A recent study suggests that it might be wise to reassess the role of calcium supplements derived from ground stones in the management of osteoporosis, because big doses of calcium supplement may be associated with an increased risk of calcium plaque accumulation in the body's arteries and thus leading to risk of heart attacks.[13]

---

[13] M. J. Bolland, A. Avenell, J. A. Baron, A. Grey, G. S. Mac Lennan, G. D. Gamble, I. R. Reid; Effect of calcium supplements on risk of myocardial infarction and cardiovascular events: meta-analysis: BMJ 2010

Maturing in the ocean, sea vegetables can remind us of our evolutionary origin – life as we know it began in the ocean from a single cell.

With this understanding in mind, eating sea vegetables can particularly help us to connect with memories and past events. The minerals in the sea vegetables are basically the molecular building blocks for rocks or stones. Rocks keep their integrity in a stable structure for a very long time – often for thousands of years. And throughout this time they are imbued with energy signatures of events occurring, which they will carry forth with them like a CD with files of information recorded upon it. Thus when eaten, minerals can activate memories in our nervous system from this life and furthermore through their energy signatures stimulate memories of events and dynamics long before we were physically born. And while these foods can reactivate history, in the deepest of terms, each moment in the body's existence is also new and freshly emerging into the world and centered right here and now.

Sea vegetables are very important for the health of our nervous system: for example, iron, which is abundant in most sea vegetables, especially red sea vegetables like dulse, is a mineral that is an important factor in producing healthy hemoglobin (the pigment contained in red blood cells) which is helping transport of oxygen throughout the body. All of our cells require oxygen to survive, but the brain (as an important part of the nervous system) is most sensitive to oxygen deprivation. Thus, an iron deficiency will reduce the blood's capacity to transport oxygen, which will greatly impact brain function.

The bio-availability of iron from sea vegetables is significant in certain sea-vegetables like arame and nori (spell nori backwards and it reads 'iron'). Iron absorption increases tremendously if Vitamin C is present in foods, as well. Nori for example contains a measurable amount of Vitamin C along with iron, which acts to increase bio-availability.

It is widely known that lack of iodine in the diet can cause brain damage and mental deficiency. All sea vegetables contain some iodine. Table salt is the current source of iodine in our western diets. At the present time most generic table salts contains sodium chloride (salt), iodine, dextrin – a form of sugar to make salt drier and easier to dispense – and various other non-natural additives. Unfortunately it is deprived of most other trace minerals except iodine.

Sea vegetables like kombu/kelp, wakame/alaria and arame are particularly concentrated sources of iodine minus the non-natural additives.

Hypothyroidism or goiters (often cause by a lack of iodine in the diet) can generally be reversed when eating sea vegetables; especially kombu, kelp, wakame or arame are known to contain concentrated sources of iodine to assist the thyroid in producing more thyroid hormone.

An adult needs approximately 0.2 milligrams of iodine daily; if you eat 1g of kombu or wakame daily (a 1.5 inch piece of kombu dry equals 1 g), you will receive the amount necessary.

In our world, where simple sugar (as in cane sugar) is pervading almost every aspect of a regular diet, I have often found that people are loosing their sense of identity and direction. Sugar is a crucial factor in creating an acidic blood condition, which in turn allows many unwelcome bacteria and virus to thrive in our system. When sugar is digested and only a minimal amount of minerals are available from the foods eaten, the body – in an attempt to keep the blood alkaline – is creating a buffer reaction, by releasing minerals from the bones into the blood stream. This pattern of eating – meaning consuming a lot of sugar over a long period of time, without adding extra minerals through diet or supplements, our bones will become de-mineralized and eventually brittle or spongy leading to osteoporosis and a variety of other diseases. Our bone marrow can be viewed metaphorically as our physical core essence. When we deplete our core essence on the physical level, it reflects often in loosing our sense of self on an emotional/mental level, as well, leading to a loss of identity.

A person exhibiting a lack or loss of identity is saying 'yes' to everything and overextending herself/himself, because of a lack of guts to say 'no' or a lack of discernment of what he or she likes or dislikes.

The minerals from sea vegetables can help to build the foundation in the body for a sense of individuality and identity along with structure and boundaries when eaten in proper amounts. And simultaneously sea vegetables are flexible and pliable, which metaphorically speaking points to a flexibility in being, in identity and boundaries, not a being that is rigid, inflexible or intolerant of other ways of doing and being.

A diet containing hardly any minerals and mostly sugars, will tend to make us emotional, forget who we are, becoming afraid of the future or creating delusional visions of the future, without the ability to simultaneously apply logic and reason to any situation given. It often gives people a false sense of connection with everything, but no sense of 'I', and hence being lost in 'mush' of emotion, that will eventually lead to a descending emotional spiral.

On the other hand, overconsumption of sea vegetables is also not advisable – just like eating too much salt is detrimental to the body. This dynamic will keep a person locked in past events or dynamics, often remembering and enumerating failures and lack of accomplishments along with being stuck in useless or at times hindering ways of doing and being – or ego dynamics along with rage at times.

Sea vegetables contain magnetic trace minerals such as iron and magnetite, which can help to give us a sense of direction in life. The center atom in each molecule of hemoglobin in the blood is iron, which makes it magnetic and direction oriented or at least subject to be aligned with electromagnetic fields in our environment – like the invisible meridians of the earth. This way we can align ourselves with the movement of Gaia, the earth, for our value fulfillment and fulfillment of our destiny. Unfortunately these days a lot of non-natural electromagnetic fields are interfering with our natural electromagnetic fields occurring in the environment from cell-phones, cell-towers, computers, refrigerators, etc. In order to align with the greater awareness of the earth, it is best to take a walk in nature, daily, best away from power-lines and cell-towers.

The iron content in sea vegetables is significant: about 2 – 10 times that of egg yolks, for example.

Some of the complex sugars in sea vegetables, called 'alginic acid', 'sodium alginate' and 'u-fucoidan'[14] among others, found in sea vegetables like kombu, wakame, arame and hiziki, have tremendous cleansing effect on our bodies. They bind with heavy metals[15] such as mercury, lead, cadmium and radioactive substances like strontium - 90, iodine - 131 in the intestines. These toxic substances are then eliminated from the body through bowl movement in the presence of the afore mentioned sea vegetables.

[14] Fillon, Mike, "Fucoidan Your Key to Wellness from the Sea"; Breakthroughs in Health, Vol. 1, Issue 3.

Maruyama H., et al. 2003. Antitumor activity and immune response of fucoidan; In Vivo.

[15] Davis, T.A. et al. 2003. Alginates bind heavy metals. Applied Biochemistry Biotechnology.

After the accident in Chernobyl, a sea vegetable called spirulina was used to help save many children from radiation poisoning.

In its natural environment, alginic acid protects the sea vegetables from the assault by bacteria and fungi, and we may conclude that it would be helpful for the same purpose in our bodies, as well.

Black color, which indicates an abundance of minerals and antioxidants in any particular food, is indicating that it can help to create a blood condition that dissolves excessive fats and proteins, as well as excessive mucous in the body. Scientists have concluded that the antioxidants in sea vegetables are promoting strong immune health and can be an important factor in helping to prevent tumors and fibroids from occurring or shrinking tumors that may already exist in the body.[16]

---

[16] Abraham, M.D., Guy E., et al. The Iodine Project: An Update 2003.

Aceves C, et al. 2005. Is iodine a gatekeeper of the integrity of the mammary gland? Journal of Mammary Gland Biology and Neoplasia.

Deville, Michel and Frederic, Trace Elements: Catalysts for Health, Switzerland, CRAO Editions 1998.

Chida, K. and Yamamoto, I; 1987. Anititumor activity of a crude fucoidan fraction prepared from the roots of kelp (Laminaria species). Kitasato Archives of Experimental Medicine.

Itoh H. et al. 1995. Immunological analysis of inhibition of lung metastases by fucoidan prepared from brown seaweed Sargassum thunbergii. Anticancer Research.

---

Many toxins in our bodies are stored in fat cells. When excessive fat cells are dissolving, it will allow the body to eliminate the toxins stored in these cells, through bowl movement, urination, deep breathing, sweating, etc.

In summary: sea vegetables improve memory, are helpful for the nervous system and brain, as well as for the circulatory system, strengthening blood quality, immune function, discharging toxins from the body. They have antibacterial and anti-tumor qualities and many have anti-coagulant substances.

In the eastern philosophy sea vegetables are classified as water energy and thus restoring organs that govern the water household in the body: kidney and bladder function, as well as reproductive organs.

Please enjoy sea vegetables as part of your regular diet. Below, please find some of my most favorite recipes - I hope you will enjoy them, as well.

# Sea Vegetable Recipes

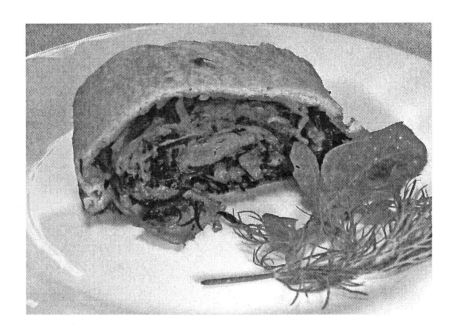

Hijiki Strudel, see page 139

# Hiziki Strudel

1/3 cup hiziki
1 cup onions, sliced into half moons
1 cup carrots, sliced into matchsticks
sesame oil
water
soy sauce
ginger juice
strudel dough (see recipe below)

Soak the hiziki in plenty of water for 30 minutes. Discard the water and if necessary cut the hijiki into small pieces. Place a heavy skillet over a medium flame and brush with sesame oil. Add the onions and sautee until they are glassy. Place the hijiki on top of the onions, then layer the carrots on top of the hijiki. Add enough water to cover the onions and bring to a boil, then simmer for approximately 15 minutes. Add a small amount of soy sauce and ginger juice and simmer a few minutes longer. Before placing this mixture on the strudel dough, let it cool a little bit.

Spread hiziki and vegetable dish evenly on the stretched dough, leaving the edges of the pastry uncovered. Roll the filled pastry into a log shape. Place the strudel on a parchment paper lined pastry sheet. Bake in a pre-heated 375 degrees oven for approximately 30 minutes or until the crust is golden brown. Remove the strudel from the oven. Serve warm.

**Strudel dough recipe:**
2 cups unbleached white flour or 1 cup unbleached white flour and 1 cup whole wheat bread flour
½ teaspoon salt
¼ cup olive oil
½ cup cold water

Combine flour and salt in a large bowl. Add the oil and mix until the flour is coated and has a pebble like consistency. Add water and knead until dough forms into a soft ball – it takes approximately 10 minutes of kneading – add a little more water if needed. Let the finished dough sit in a cool place for a minimum of ½ hour, then stretch dough out by pulling it from the center into all directions equally into a very thin layer. You can roll the dough, however a rolled dough is generally not as thin as a hand stretched dough.

# Light Lemon Pudding

4 cups apple juice
pinch of sea salt
2 tablespoons agar flakes
¼ cup rice syrup or maple syrup
2 – 3 tablespoons kuzu, diluted in 3 – 4 tablespoons water
2 tablespoons lemon juice
1 – 2 teaspoons organic lemon zest
mint leaves or almond slivers for garnish

Place apple juice, salt, agar flakes and syrup of your choice into a saucepan. Bring to a boil and simmer until the agar flakes are completely dissolved. Add the diluted kuzu gradually, while stirring constantly to prevent lumping. Simmer until the pudding thickens. Add lemon juice and zest; stir gently and remove from heat.

Pour into individual dessert cups to let it set. Garnish with mint leaves or almond slivers.

## Arame with Dried Daikon and Carrots and Onions

½ cup arame, rinsed
½ cup dried daikon, soaked for 20 minutes and cut into smaller strands
1 – 2 onions cut into thin half moons
1 – 2 carrots cut into matchsticks
sesame oil
soy sauce
water

Heat a skillet over a medium flame and brush with sesame oil. Add onions and sauté until they become glassy. Then layer the arame on top of the onions, then the dried daikon and finally the onions. Add water (and/or use dried daikon soaking water) to cover half of the ingredients. Once the water comes to a boil, cover and turn flame down to a low simmer.

Cook for approximately 20 minutes. Uncover and season with soy sauce and continue to cook for another 5 minutes (without a cover) or until all the liquid in the skillet has been evaporated.

## Noodle-Vegetable Aspic with Pumpkinseed Dressing

1 package (8 ounces) of udon noodles
3 inch long strip of kombu, sliced into very thin strips
4 dried shiitake, soaked and sliced
4 cups of water
3 - 4 tablespoons of soysauce or tamari or to taste
1 teaspoon fresh ginger juice
1 medium carrot, cut into flowerets
½ cup corn, fresh or frozen
¼ cup scallions or chives, finely sliced
4 tablespoons agar flakes

Cook the noodles (follow the instructions on the package) and drain them well. Transfer the drained noodles into a deep casserole dish.

Place kombu, shiitake and water into a saucepan and bring to a boil. Reduce the flame to medium low, add carrot, summer squash and agar flakes and simmer for approximately 10 minutes or until the agar flakes are completely dissolved. Add shoyu to taste and simmer 3 to 5 minutes longer. Turn the flame off and add ginger juice and scallions or chives.

Pour the vegetable broth with the vegetables over the noodles and set aside to cool and gel. Once it is set, cut into slices and serve. Garnish with parsley and pumpkinseed dressing.

## Pumpkinseed Dressing
## ½ cup of pumpkinseeds

2 umeboshi plums
spring water
¼ cup finely cut parsley, scallions or chives

Sort, wash and dry roast pumpkin seeds in a skillet.

Grind to a paste in the suribachi (grinding bowl) or grind in a blender. Remove the pit from the umeboshi plums, finely chop the plums and grind to a paste with the seeds, also adding the parsley, scallions or chives. Add water to obtain desired consistency.

# Quick Nori Cucumber Salad

2 sheets of nori, torn or cut into small pieces
½ cucumber, sliced into thin half moons
1 tablespoon of sweet rice vinegar
1 tablespoon of water or shiitake-kombu soaking water
1 teaspoon of soy sauce or tamari
1 good size pinch of sea salt

Soak the nori for 3 minutes in cold water, then squeeze the nori out and discard the soaking water. Set the nori aside.

Mix the cucumber slices with the sea salt and press for approximately 5 minutes until the cucumber releases some of its water. Squeeze excess water out of the cucumber and discard water.

Prepare a marinade with the rice vinegar, water or shiitake-kombu soaking water and soy sauce. Place the nori and cucumber into the marinade and mix well. Serve room temperature.

## Green Tea Kanten

2 cups water
1 - 2 teaspoons green tea powder
2 tablespoons agar-agar flakes
½ cup of rice syrup or to taste
pinch of sea salt

Place the water and agar agar flakes into a saucepan, with a pinch of sea salt. Bring the water to a boil, then reduce the flame to low, add the rice syrup and simmer until flakes are dissolved (about 2 – 5 minutes). Stir occasionally. Turn the flame off and let agar/water mixture sit for 3 – 4 minutes before vigorously stirring in the green tea powder.

Pour into individual dessert bowls to set.
When jelled serve as is, or with roasted, black sesame seeds for garnish; or serve with fresh fruit topping of your choice.

# Nori Condiment

5 – 6 sheets of nori, torn or cut into one-inch pieces
or smaller
water
1 – 3 teaspoons of soysauce or tamari or to taste
1 teaspoon umeboshi paste
1 – 2 teaspoons of fresh ginger juice or to taste

Place the nori strips into a saucepan and cover with
water. Dilute the umeboshi paste with a small
amount of water and add into the saucepan. Bring the
mixture to a boil, then simmer covered for
approximately 10 minutes, adding water if necessary.
Add soysauce or tamari and ginger juice to taste and
simmer another 5 minutes. Serve immediately or
store in a glass jar for up to 3 days.

Variation: add dried, soaked shiitake or add rice
syrup.


# Wakame with Fu and Onions

½ package fu, soaked 10 minutes and sliced
½ cup wakame, soaked and sliced
2 cups onions, sliced in thin half moons
3 – 4 tablespoons roasted tahini (sesamebutter)
½ - 1 cup water
soy sauce or tamari to taste

Saute the onions, wakame and fu in a skillet with a little water. Dilute the tahini with water and season with soysauce to taste. Once the onions are glassy and the wakame is soft, mix the diluted tahini into the sauté and cook for another few minutes with a cover over a low flame.

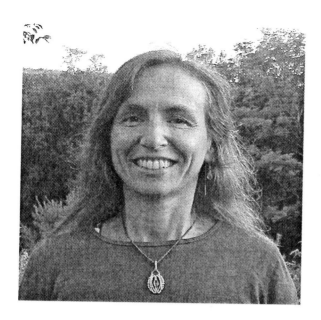

## About Myself:

Realizing the complex interconnections between body, mind and spirit, I know from my own experience that it is possible to improve one's health and to deepen the quality of all experiences in life. It is my intent to share this knowledge and wisdom of this path for better health and vitality to the best of my ability, so that we may pursue our most passionate dreams in life with harm to none.

I was born in Rendsburg, Germany – a small town on the Baltic Sea, close to Denmark. I love the sea. The sea is always doing what she does, no matter whether there is worldwide peace or worldwide crisis. The salt scent in the air and the regular change from low tide to high tide has always felt comforting. When I was 6 years old, we moved to the border of the Netherlands, where I lived with my family until I moved to the US in 1992.

I began studying Macrobiotics in Germany in 1985 (still a teenager then) as a natural extension of my personal studies pertaining to the nature of consciousness and the knowledge that everything is and has consciousness - even though it may be very alien to our sense of consciousness. I believe there to be an innate relationship between all portions of nature, as all is consciousness. Our natural phenomena - such as the weather - represent the inner reality of our feelings collectively, while objects and things are 'thought events' and thoughts are just as much nature events as are rain or wind.

I decided to study Food Science and Dietetics at the University of Muenster along with studying Macrobiotics and conscious creation to be able to combine the Eastern and Western approach.

Edward Esko, a teacher for Macrobiotics at the Kushi Institute in Becket, Massachusetts, for whom I had translated at a Macrobiotic Leadership/Career Training Seminar in Germany in 1991, invited me to visit the Kushi Institute. I happily took the opportunity after finishing my studies, intending to stay for only 6 months. Well, 6 months have become several decades now and I am still here, and happy to be here.

Since then I have taught and counseled Macrobiotics and other Body-Mind-Spirit related subjects such as Meditation, Chanting, Tai Chi, Qi Gong and intuitive counseling in the United States and in Europe for over 25 years now.

I never experienced any serious health challenge, until the summer of 2011. That summer I suddenly developed an unusual inability to be outside during the day exposed to the sun. If I weeded my garden for more than 20 minutes while the sun was shining, I would develop a headache and sometimes feel quite nauseous. In previous years I could stay outside all day without any problems. Initially I attributed this to the fact that perhaps the ozone layer was getting thinner and more harmful rays from the sun were reaching the earth's surface as my son had shared with me how the ozone layer is becoming precariously thin in the Northeastern United States these days through his studies of Environmental Sciences at the College.

After a particularly busy summer, in terms of work, I traveled with my son to Germany to visit my family towards the end of August. I began developing a stiff neck during the flight and this symptom didn't quite leave for the whole duration of my visit in Germany. The weather was cold and damp in Germany and even inside my mother's house it always felt uncomfortably cold and moist, so I didn't pay too much attention to this irksome symptom, partially also because I hadn't seen my family in a long time and was somewhat focused on them, not myself.

After a two-week stay in Germany it was time for our flight back to the US. The flight was uneventful. However, by the time we arrived in Boston, my neck was becoming very painful, in fact so painful, that I couldn't move my neck at all: when I leaned my head back against the seat cushion in the airport (our ride home from Boston was 4 hours delayed, because of a miscommunication) I had to manually lift my head with my hands into an upright position, because it was impossible for me to do it otherwise.

I was so glad to be home after 28 hours of travel, but now I was facing another dilemma: I couldn't get myself undressed to take a shower or go to bed. My neck, including part of my upper spine, shoulders and upper arms were so painful, that I could not even lift my arms any longer. I had to ask my son to help me get undressed. I knew I was in serious trouble then.

I made an appointment with a doctor, but the doctor couldn't see me until a month later. In the meantime I tried to diagnose myself, typing the symptoms into search engines on the internet and using my macrobiotic diagnostic skills. I didn't come up with any clear diagnosis of my problem – I even asked other experienced macrobiotic counselors and health practitioners and they were not able to pinpoint any particular condition or disorder, either. My symptoms had disappeared by the time of the scheduled visit with the doctor - my neck and shoulders were perfectly fine again. The doctor suggested a general blood test, which returned all within normal ranges, in other words I seemed healthy.

A week after the doctor's visit my right knee swell up to the size of a volley-ball – I didn't know that any body part could swell up that much; it was extremely painful. I scheduled another appointment with the doctor – and again I had to wait 3 weeks to see the doctor. Meanwhile the swelling lasted 3 days with such intense pain, I could not sleep, then subsided. One week later, my left knee began to swell, then my left hand, all with excruciating pain. Realizing that the swellings and pain kept migrating with arthritis-like symptoms I was able to narrow my own diagnosis. I walked into the doctor's office armed with my conclusions and a request for at least one test I wanted to be checked out for: lyme disease. The doctor agreed and also suggested checking for parvo virus and rheumatoid arthritis (which I really didn't think it was, but some of the symptoms were consistent with the disease).

Three days later I received a phone call from my doctor late in the evening: she told me that the results were in: I had lyme disease, which is supposedly contracted by a tick bite – I never had a tick bite that I was aware of and thus never had any of the earmark signs (bulls eye ring around bite, swelling, etc.). My doctor was shocked by the results because the test showed that I must have had the lyme disease for a long time, perhaps 2 years or so, because the results for the antibodies my body had created were off the charts. The doctor commented that she had never seen anyone with a test result like mine, and people she had seen, who had high levels of antibodies (but not close to where my levels were) were completely incapacitated by fatigue, joint pain, debilitating arthritis like symptoms in many parts of the body, mental fog, migraines and other obscure symptoms that would leave a person unable to work for weeks, even months. I hardly developed any symptoms in comparison, which I attribute to eating a well rounded macrobiotic diet. And I realized, that I had only developed symptoms during the summer of 2011 after a particularly emotionally stressful period of time in my life: I just had closed a business, in which I was involved in for 3 years with 2 partners, who also used to be my friends. At the closing of the business we had enough money to pay off all outstanding accounts, however my partners – a married couple, outvoted me in paying off the outstanding accounts and instead made investments with the money for themselves, because they were paranoid that the world was going to 'end' and they needed to stockpile food and other items for their own survival. The world didn't fall apart and the creditors began calling them. When the bills kept coming they asked me begin paying for them - I was outraged! I talked to a lawyer, but decided to try to reason with the couple first on my own before choosing to take the route of the law process. I met them at their house. For the purpose of having peace with them, after quite some back and forth of arguments, we had almost reached an agreement, and the wife of the couple was going to draft an agreement. I agreed with the stipulation that I would be able to show this document to my lawyer before signing it. She adamantly insisted that I had to sign the document without showing it to my lawyer or anyone else. At that moment an angel-like being appeared in front of me and I knew in that instant that this was the wrong choice. It felt like a manipulation for their personal benefit and power over me. I then got up and left their house.

I then involved a lawyer to sort out the unfortunate situation; the proceedings were drawn out but ended favorably.

However, during this stressful time, I often wondered how I could have been so stupid not to see this particular dynamic coming. In hindsight I can clearly see how this pattern of self-loathing and attacking myself mentally and emotionally was enough to weaken my immune system to let the lyme spiroketes become active in my system, whereas before, they likely were present, but could not become active, because my immune system was strong, having been built up by eating mostly unprocessed, macrobiotic foods for a long time. Only when I began systematically questioning and doubting myself, did I undermine my immune function.

The journey back to full health took a bit longer than I wished it to be – a full 6 months to recover, but considering the doctor's distressed surprise at the severity of my lyme test results, I was never in really bad shape – although by my standards I wasn't feeling well.

During the time of recovery, I was extremely sensitive to many foods, even many good quality macrobiotic foods. Wheat or barley in any form didn't agree with me, neither did any sweets or fruits, spices, excess salt or excess fish. On the other hand, I craved sea vegetables, especially arame and hijiki, burdock, kale and long fermented pickles more than any other time in my life. I am grateful to have such strong allies in healing!

Ever since one of my houseplants had begun communicating with me (in the past I had heard that people talk to plants, but I never knew they could talk back!) I have understood that all plants have consciousness. Most often I ask the (consciousness of the ) vegetables I prepare for food to meld with my consciousness for mutual benefit. In that process I have often found an immediate sense of agreement and wellbeing and a positive surge in my energy level.

The physical body reacts to our emotional, physical and mental input of the present moment. Worrying about unfavorable situations of the past or future confuses the body's mechanisms and undermines healthy functions of the body. While disadvantageous circumstances may exist in our life, it is always helpful to remember that auspicious and favorable events take place far more often than the negative ones, otherwise the world would long have ceased to exist in my opinion.

And so during my healing journey it became abundantly clear that I needed to change my ways of doing and being – and while it is never a perfect process, it was important for me to remember often enough to stop the self loathing, and instead rejoicing in who I am and in my abilities, so that this new way of doing and being became more deeply ingrained than the previous neural pathway of beating myself up.

Every morning I meditate and chant and most evenings I take a short time to do so, as well, so that I set the intent for the day and/or night and feel the energy of love, appreciation and gratitude coursing through me. These energy signatures clearly make a difference in my daily outlook on life. Also exercise is an important aspect – especially light to moderate exercise in a natural environment, like going for a walk in nature, etc. While we are healthy, we may never notice how deeply walking on the grass can affect the body, but when we are on a healing journey, the increased sense of energy and wellbeing from such practices is tremendous and not to be overlooked.

I know humanity is standing at a crossroads and there is more than one path to choose. However, I wish to participate with you in a world where we innately know of our connection with each other and our loving presence radiates with joy and peace; and our fulfillment of our greatest potentials is attained, while simultaneously also furthering the greatest potential of each other human being and portion of our world and universe.